Praise for

Counseling People with Early-Stage Alzheimer's Disease: A Powerful Process of Transformation

"Robyn Yale's framework of clinical counseling for people with early memory loss . . . provides an outstanding model. The unique concerns of people with early dementia . . . need to be dealt with sensitively and expertly, and this book gives counselors the tools they need to do just that."

> —**Ginny Helms,** *Vice President of Chapter Services & Public Policy, Alzheimer's Association, Georgia Chapter*

"This important book fills a critical gap in caring for the person in a culture where emphasis is often placed on the disease. Yale's advice is grounded in years of personal experience with hundreds of people with early-stage dementia."

> —**Bruce L. Miller, M.D.,** *Director, University of California–San Francisco Memory and Aging Center*

"This book will be invaluable for all those engaged in, or embarking on, the process of counseling people with early-stage dementia. It should also be read by anyone in contact with people who have early-stage dementia, as it provides the best guide I have yet come across to understanding what it is like to experience early-stage dementia and how to respond in a helpful and positive way. Yale's passion and commitment to helping people to live well with dementia shine through on every page, and make reading this book an exciting and deeply inspiring experience."

> —**Linda Clare, Ph.D. ,** *Professor of Clinical Psychology and Neuropsychology, Bangor University (U.K.)*

"Drawing on the strengths of many therapeutic styles compatible for work with early-stage individuals, this book provides a solid guide through the many challenges experienced by those diagnosed. The strengths of the person diagnosed and the therapist are honored throughout the process. . . . "

> —**Judy Filippoff, MSW,** *Early Stage Program Coordinator, Alzheimer's Association, Northern California and Northern Nevada*

"In this pioneering work, Yale offers a dynamic, real-world, and relationship-based model for counseling persons with dementia that embraces the invaluable principles of evolution and resilience. Her framework is grounded in many years of listening to the concerns and needs of persons with memory loss with both empathy and respect, and through her wise, engaging, and informative writing, she reveals how both the client and counselor can be transformed by this practice."

—*Lisa Snyder, LCSW, author,* Speaking Our Minds: What It's Like to Have Alzheimer's *and* Living Your Best with Early-Stage Alzheimer's

"This text is essential reading if we are to ensure that our response to dementia is a positive, transformative one! . . . [This is] a stimulating wealth of knowledge that makes a fascinating read."

—*Professor Heather Wilkinson, Co-director, Centre for Research on Families and Relationships, University of Edinburgh (U.K.)*

"Presented in a fresh and original style . . . Robyn Yale provides an excellent foundation for understanding the special issues that people with early dementia face, and details a clear, compelling model for one-on-one clinical counseling based on her many years of experience."

—*Suzette Binford, Programs Director, Alzheimer's Association, Georgia Chapter*

"[This] well-written and practical book captures the multidimensional experience of people living with Alzheimer's disease and challenges professionals to expand their repertoire of therapeutic interventions for those facing this life-altering experience."

—*Darby Morhardt, MSW, LCSW, Research Associate Professor and Director of Education, Cognitive Neurology and Alzheimer's Disease Center, Northwestern University Feinberg School of Medicine*

"Another excellent resource from Robyn Yale . . . [She] takes readers through every step . . . as she discusses counseling in the early stages."

—*Sam Fazio, PhD, author of* The Enduring Self in People with Alzheimer's *and co-author of* Rethinking Alzheimer's Care

"This book represents a breakthrough in the development of the person-centred approach in dementia care. . . . [It] has a welcome practical focus, . . . reflecting the importance of tangible, attainable changes within the context of a difficult and potentially overwhelming condition. Empowerment is a key concept."

—*Bob Woods, Professor of Clinical Psychology of Older People, Bangor University (U.K.)*

Also by Robyn Yale

Developing Support Groups for Individuals with Early-Stage Alzheimer's Disease: Planning, Implementation, and Evaluation

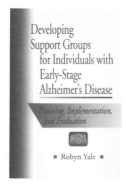

"Robyn Yale's early-stage support group model has been replicated worldwide, and this excellent book provides you with everything you need to develop a success-ful program. Even experienced professionals and support group facilitators can glean valuable information, and it can be referred to as needed for creative ideas, problem solving, and insightful reminders. I consider it a must-have reference on the library shelf of anyone working in the field of early-stage dementia. . . ."
—Lisa Snyder, LCSW, Alzheimer's Disease Research Center,
University of California–San Diego

For more information, visit http://www.healthpropress.com

Counseling People with Early-Stage Alzheimer's Disease

A Powerful Process of Transformation

by

Robyn Yale, LCSW

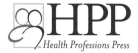

HPP
Health Professions Press

Baltimore • London • Sydney

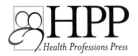

Health Professions Press, Inc.
Post Office Box 10624
Baltimore, Maryland 21285-0624

www.healthpropress.com

Interior and cover designs by Mindy Dunn.
Cover photo: Copyright © 2013 by David Assmann.
Typeset by Barton Matheson Willse & Worthington, Baltimore, Maryland.
Manufactured in the United States of America by Versa Press, East Peoria, Illinois.

Developed and written by Robyn Yale, LCSW, in collaboration with and funded by the Alzheimer's Association, Georgia Chapter. This project was supported in part by grant number 90A10034/02, from the U.S. Administration on Aging, U.S. Department of Health and Human Services in conjunction with the Georgia Department of Human Services/Division of Aging Services. Grantees undertaking projects under government sponsorship are encouraged to express freely their findings and conclusions. Points of view or opinions do not, therefore, necessarily represent official Administration on Aging policy.

Library of Congress Cataloging-in-Publication Data

Yale, Robyn, author.
  Counseling people with early-stage Alzheimer's disease : a powerful process of transformation / by Robyn Yale.
     p. ; cm.
  Includes bibliographical references and index.
  ISBN 978-1-938870-07-1 (pbk.)
  I. Title.
  [DNLM: 1. Alzheimer Disease. 2. Counseling—methods. 3. Professional-Patient Relations. WT 155]
  RC523
  616.8ʼ3106—dc23
                                                                              2013026934

British Library Cataloguing in Publication data are available from the British Library.

This book is dedicated to the courageous professionals in the early-stage Alzheimer's field, and the people with dementia who inspire us all.

Contents

About the Author

Robyn Yale, LCSW, is a licensed clinical social worker with more than 30 years of experience in the fields of aging and Alzheimer's disease. In 1986, she pioneered the innovative *early-stage support group*, which gave people with Alzheimer's disease an opportunity to talk with one another and better understand the illness. This experience informed her belief that information and support is as critical for people with dementia as it is for those facing any other illness. In addition to authoring the book *Developing Support Groups for Individuals with Early-Stage Alzheimer's Disease: Planning, Implementation, and Evaluation* (1995, Health Professions Press), she was among the first to promote early-stage awareness and services and facilitate collaboration among professionals around the world in this area.

Yale's group model has been widely replicated internationally through her book and training presentations in more than one hundred cities spanning five continents. Her teaching aims to give clarity to early-stage issues, and courage to professionals who want to do this fascinating work. Her work received the national MindAlert Award from the American Society on Aging. She also developed a model of memory loss support groups for residents of assisted living that has been implemented in many communities.

Yale works as an independent consultant and is based in San Francisco, California.

Prologue

The Power of Transformation

This is a tale about the power of transformation. Tales express rich metaphors that universalize the human condition. They contain themes, archetypes, central characters, unfolding stories, and a quest from which we glean life lessons. They illuminate the challenges we all face, and remind us to access our own inner strengths. What follows is a true story of self-discovery, which transforms people with early dementia as well as practitioners.

The alchemy of transformation also affects the dementia care field, and ultimately brings about stunning social change. You will find that these threads are woven throughout our tale. They are represented by the terms "revolution" and "evolution."

Setting the Context: Revolution and Evolution

*Like art, revolutions come from combining what exists
into what has never existed before.*

—Gloria Steinem

People with early-stage dementia (PWESD)* due to Alzheimer's disease (AD) or related disorders must valiantly fight an uphill battle against their condition. They

---

*The acronym PWESD is used throughout the book to refer to both singular and plural; that is, "person with early-stage dementia" as well as "people with early-stage dementia."

1

are not typically armored with individualized education and support to cope with the enormous challenges. Many become isolated and marginalized. Counseling empowers people to become fierce warriors: by understanding and coming to terms with the illness, while also making healthy adaptations to it. The heart of the struggle—and the key element for victory—is the relationship with the counselor. When people are offered the opportunity to discuss their situation rather than despair and give up, heroic transformation can occur. PWESD attain hope and valuable insights, uncover existing strengths, and become fortified with new opportunities for meaning, connection, and contribution in their lives.

The field of dementia care has been radically altered by both revolution and evolution in the last few decades. Remarkable progress has seismically shifted the predominant view that nothing can be done for diagnosed persons, as they, along with their family and professional care partners, have refuted negative stereotypes, reaffirmed their "personhood," and blazed a trail to form many innovative programs. PWESD are now often educators and advocates at professional conferences, legislative hearings, and community events, and are more likely to be acknowledged and included in decisions affecting their lives. The media still typically focus on AD as an end point for people. But there are now also more enlightened reports about those courageously facing their diagnosis, adapting to it, and carrying on with previous or new work or other activities for as long as possible.

Synthesizing various definitions, revolution involves sweeping change, within a relatively short period of time, in the way of thinking about or visualizing something. It challenges the social order, ideology, culture, and policy as well as organizational structures and systems. Evolution, on the other hand, is the more gradual process of developing into a different and usually better form, over a longer period of time. Applying these concepts here, we could say that, having begun to fundamentally reform perceptions of people with dementia and the way we serve them, there is still a long way to go, and it is an incremental, ongoing effort.

Project Partners

My own perspective has always been rooted in activism. I've been in the Alzheimer's field for over 30 years, and I developed what's been credited as the first early-stage support group model in 1986. Later, I tailored the approach further to offset the stigma and secrecy about living with dementia in residential care settings. These support groups help PWESD share their feelings and experiences, and it struck me that they were learning how to live rather than waiting to die with the disease. I have trained others nationally and internationally so that the groups would become more widely available, and received a MindAlert award from the American Society on Aging for pioneering this work. In those early years, I provided an international newsletter to professionals, facilitating the exchange of information, support, and resources. But even more importantly, others became motivated by the same experience that I had: learning *from* PWESD that many are willing and able to talk about and learn to cope with this condition as one would with any other, and as you or I might in the same situation. This new end of the field took on an extraordinary momentum of its own, with many agencies creating programs to meet the multidimensional recreational, social, educational, and vocational needs that exist at this early point in the disease course.

Throughout my career, I've also done individual counseling with PWESD, which informed the foundation of this book. In 2010 when I was contacted by the Georgia Chapter of the Alzheimer's Association to consult on a pilot project around clinical counseling for people with early-stage dementia, I was most interested. This was part of a larger grant the Chapter had received from the U.S. Administration on Aging, which aimed to have staff better identify people with early-stage AD, help them understand the disease and its progression, and use psychotherapeutic and other techniques to relieve distress and promote well-being. The Chapter approached me with a central question: How can we help people cope with early dementia? They asked me to develop an effective intervention around this for training and implementation with their regional Area Agencies on Aging (AAAs).

I was delighted to accept the invitation to collaborate, and I applaud Ginny Helms, Suzette Binford, and Susan Formby of the Chapter, as well as Cliff Burt of the Georgia Division of Aging Services, for their vision and determination to venture into this relatively new terrain. Working with them has been exceptional, as they were equipped with a wealth of knowledge and excellent clinical experience. The Georgia Chapter is one of the more solid and well established in the early-stage area, having long done support groups along with social and art programs for PWESD. They were just the right professionals to take on clinical counseling, and this sparked a creative synergy that helped to articulate, refine, and bring the model to life over our 3 years of consultation together. I'm also pleased about their partnership with the AAAs. Janice Adams (Central Savannah River Area Regional Commission) joined Suzette and Susan in taking on the counseling with a lot of heart and valuable insights. Since the role of AAAs also includes supporting, connecting, and offering resources to families, counseling in this setting provides another potential entry point for engaging and serving PWESD and their care partners sooner along the continuum of dementia care.

The pilot project also had an evaluation component, which was conducted in collaboration with Beth Fuller and Kristi Fuller of the Georgia Health Policy Center.

Enhancing the Field

Generally speaking, there are not many clinicians providing this service—or even thinking about it, for that matter. Few have the knowledge or skills required to offer it, even within the mental health or dementia care fields. There has been no systematized, replicable model of counseling for PWESD, and few books or workshops are available on the subject for professionals. In fact, in the past, people were routinely not told that their diagnosis was Alzheimer's disease. Now they are more frequently told, but not usually provided with much hope or direction afterward. The increasing prevalence of diagnosis in the early stages will result in many people having the capacity to face their circumstances proactively, as one would with any other illness. And the tsunami of people projected to be diagnosed in the coming years makes the development of interventions to help them cope effectively a critical need.

Early-stage Alzheimer's services that now exist include support groups, socialization and outings, memory enhancement, and art programs. In consulting with PWESD and families it is common for professionals to focus on practical and planning issues, but the emotional piece is typically overlooked because it is difficult. This counseling model is unusual in that it makes the process of understanding and coming to terms with a diagnosis of dementia a central cornerstone of what is offered. It can occur in many settings, including Alzheimer's organizations, diagnostic clinics, assisted living and other residential care facilities, mental health centers, and private practice offices (e.g., geriatric care managers, social workers, therapists, psychologists, psychiatrists). And it can be provided in either a short-term or long-term format, depending upon available resources. Those who provide the service, then, will acquire state-of-the-art, very specialized, and sorely needed expertise.

Clinical counseling adds to the range of what is offered, occurring one-to-one, and recognizing that different PWESD prefer different interventions. The more that PWESD and their care partners can access counseling, the more we expand our early-stage service infrastructure, and refine its culture.

Structure and Outcome

Our tale centers around a new Framework For Coping With Early Dementia that integrates the many emotional, practical, and lifestyle issues faced at this point in the illness. The protocol identifies an individual's challenges, sets goals to address them in counseling, and evaluates progress toward these goals after intervening. Eighteen areas are covered, including identity and self-esteem, resilience, relating to and educating others, stress management, and many others. Family caregivers also attend part of the counseling sessions, to facilitate a sense of partnership and teamwork.

The results of the pilot project in Georgia indicated that professionals and clients were all excited and positive about the counseling service. Each PWESD is different, and each has a unique emotional response upon learning their diagnosis. But all were similarly grateful for having someone to talk with personally, rather than being abandoned by a doctor who declared they had Alzheimer's disease and simply said, "Come back again in six months." PWESD said that they benefited in such ways as processing feelings, understanding the disease, better managing their symptoms, and anticipating the future.

Counselors were also asked to evaluate the program, and described profound learning as they developed new skills, competencies, and perspectives. It is clear that counseling can evoke a radical shift in how professionals regard PWESD, and how PWESD view themselves. And professionals offering counseling to PWESD are greatly enriched by the fascinating experience.

Universal and Unique Struggles

Revolution and evolution can each occur on both an individual and a societal level. Revolution can be tumultuous and shake things up, or it can be peaceful. As a nation, we are battling Alzheimer's with biomedical research advances. In our agencies and practices, we are advocating new approaches. Now, think for a moment about how we all evolve throughout our lives, in the process of knowing and becoming ourselves. Life entails crises, illness, and other circumstances that spur personal growth as we marshal the forces of inner strength and outer resources necessary to survive. Illuminating the dark corners of our fears, we strive to overcome the enormity of our emotional and tactical hurdles. Individuals bring their own equipment of experience, attitudes, and coping skills to reconcile with whatever befalls them.

All of this is equally true for people with dementia, but even more poignant. As professional counselors, we can help them mine their characters and difficult situations with determination and fortitude. The task is as simple as a kind presence, yet as complex as the deepest spiritual journey. We can't, of course, remove the adversity—but we can offer a place to metabolize it, and a measure of healing.

The counselor is an ally who steadies and sustains PWESD at a time of terror and anguish. Being with people with dementia in this way can stir up our own issues and vulnerability. It also requires wearing a variety of hats. It takes our tenacity to sit and listen; our creativity to seek solutions where they are possible; and our versatility in assuming a number of other roles. We facilitate contemplation, but also action. At various times, depending upon the client, we may be a confidante, companion, coach, care planner, career adviser, consultant, conflict resolution manager, and even a communications specialist!

Putting their trust and faith in you as a counselor, PWESD learn how to cultivate the same in themselves. And truly, if they can be so brave, then we must too. Our unfolding story about various aspects of the inner and outer life of PWESD is multihued. I'm honored and happy to have your interest, and I trust that this book will give you the courage, tools, and template to venture forth.

A Few Last Metaphors

One additional definition of "revolution" is that of turning on an axis. The dementia care field revolves around the enterprise of scientific discovery. Advances in diagnostic and treatment methods are evolving, but progress is slow. Medications are helpful to some people, for some time, but thus far do not cure AD, and do not work for everyone. Even if they did, as with any other illness, amassing additional armor is a necessity and a right. This counseling model and book are dedicated to that transformative revolutionary and evolutionary feat.

CHAPTER 1

Introduction

Looking Back and Forward

Inspiration and Aspiration

After I got the diagnosis of Alzheimer's from my doctor, I felt lost.
I didn't feel like I could really talk to my family and friends about it.
Some of them were too upset, some I think just didn't want to face it.
It was a very lonely time for me.

This sentiment is increasingly common amongst the many people who find themselves newly diagnosed with early dementia. Diagnosis can occur at varying points in the progression of the disease. One may be close to, already into, or way beyond even the middle stages. But with the increasing focus on early detection in recent years, more people are being evaluated at the beginning stage of the process.

Traditionally, services like care consultation, counseling, and support groups have targeted family members more than people who have dementia. In the general aging field, people with early-stage dementia (PWESD) don't often come to the attention of local senior and mental health agencies, who may also not know how or want to work with them. Organizations specialized in Alzheimer's disease (AD) have more services than they used to for PWESD, but individual counseling is rarely available.

Thus, PWESD typically have nowhere to turn for direction, guidance, or even an outlet to express their feelings, which may include anger, grief, frustration, worry, and fear. Well-meaning family members may unintentionally further isolate the diagnosed person out of concern that the condition shouldn't be acknowledged or discussed. The label of AD usually provokes an expectation of diminishment and incapacity rather than recognizing the vitality and capability that are still possible. As a result, PWESD are often denied the opportunity to honor and nourish the fullest potential of the self that remains within them.

Historical Perspective

The stigma and resistance around dementia used to be even more entrenched than they are now. The prevailing belief was that people shouldn't know that their diagnosis was dementia, since they couldn't understand or talk about it. Surrounded by mysterious silence, who wouldn't become immobilized by thoughts of decline and death?

A grassroots "movement" has evolved since the mid-1980s to challenge and reframe this paradigm. Early-stage support groups were developed[1] for people to share what they have in common, as happens universally in support groups around other illnesses or issues. What we (in the field) heard was, "I'm still a person; and I'm still here." While some PWESD do deny or lack insight into their condition, many are willing and able to face it as they strive to understand and cope with it. Professionals learned that when PWESD reach out to one another and to their families, it helps them live full and meaningful lives for as long as possible.

We now know that deeply listening and respectfully talking to PWESD raises awareness, opens possibilities, and paves new avenues for strengthened relationships, pleasurable activity, and purposeful engagement. New talents can be discovered and previous roles redefined. For example, many PWESD have written and spoken publicly about their experiences, found artistic and other creative outlets, and served on committees and boards of Alzheimer's organizations. Of course, not all PWESD take on such high-profile projects. But any who choose to align with the truth of what is happening rather than avoid confronting it begin an immense and heroic quest that will take them someplace different, even if it is completely private.

Paving New Ground Together

As stereotypes were challenged, new ground was forged between PWESD, their families, and professionals, and the strides made fueled organizational developments across the United States and around the world. National and international AD organizations began seeking the input of PWESD to develop federal plans, policies, and materials geared toward them, instead of only toward their families. For example, Alzheimer's Disease International's "Charter of Principles" proclaimed that all people with dementia have worth and dignity and should have access to support; and that professionals must understand their perspective in order to provide effective care and services.[2] Another effort occurred in 2007–08 when town hall meetings were held across the United States by the national Alzheimer's Association to more formally ask PWESD what they want and need. The compelling testimony reaffirmed what professionals had been learning in early-stage support groups and other interactions with PWESD in the preceding years. What they were looking for included

- learning what to expect and how to cope with the disease,

- remaining included in decisions and activities to the extent possible, and

- being heard, seen, and respected as viable, contributing members of society.[3]

The Georgia Chapter held one of these forums and became motivated to initiate what you are now reading. As described earlier, they were concerned that, while progress has been made in the number and variety of programs available to PWESD, few settings anywhere offer one-to-one clinical counseling. Our collaboration resulted in a body of work that can be easily replicated by others. It may still be commonly assumed that PWESD are unable to benefit from counseling, but the collective wisdom of those in the early dementia field is that not only is it appropriate, but it's very much needed; and as you will see, also quite feasible.

Previewing the Framework for Coping with Early Dementia

While it's necessary to acknowledge the significant losses that accompany dementia, diagnosed individuals don't have to be characterized as "victims" and "sufferers." Working through emotions, adapting to practical circumstances, and retaining autonomy about lifestyle preferences as much as one is able to fosters resilience and encourages people to move forward with their lives. These three interrelated domains are the cornerstones of coping effectively with early dementia, and are the heart of this counseling approach. You will find that an issue arising in any one area will impact, and be impacted by, the other two. Each of the three main areas is further broken down into six elements as depicted in Figure 1.1, which we will be exploring in more detail. An integrated version of the Framework for Coping with Early Dementia can be found in the next chapter (Figure 2.3), and will be used thereafter.

Two Critical Ingredients

There are two critical ingredients required for this intervention.

First, it is important to note here that not all PWESD are good candidates for counseling. A well-refined process to assess and select those most likely to benefit from it is described in Chapter 10. Necessary characteristics include being aware of one's condition, being willing and able to talk about it, and wanting to be in

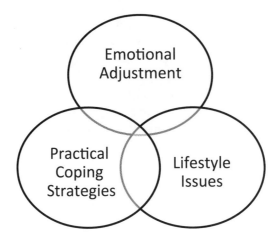

EMOTIONAL ADJUSTMENT	PRACTICAL COPING STRATEGIES	LIFESTYLE ISSUES
Acceptance of Condition	Stress Management	Social and Vocational Activities
Existential Issues	Memory Aids	Future Planning
Identity	Communication Techniques	Family Relationships
Expressing Feelings	Physical Wellness	Asking For/Accepting Help
Resilience	Cognitive Exercise	Service Utilization
Relating to Others	Support System	Problem Solving: Safety Issues

Figure 1.1. Three domains and eighteen elements of the Framework for Coping with Early Dementia (Copyright © 2011, by Robyn Yale)

counseling. There we will also discuss the skills needed to engage and communicate with PWESD about their diagnosis before the intake process can even begin.

Second, counselors must be well credentialed, as described in Chapter 4. This includes a relevant degree, a specialized mix of social work and mental health/counseling backgrounds, and dementia care experience. Early-stage training and ongoing clinical supervision are also essential.

These elements, along with the power of the counseling relationship, are key to achieving a successful therapeutic process.

Traditional Counseling: Differences and Similarities

While this counseling model is new and innovative, counseling PWESD is both similar to and different from "traditional" counseling, or counseling people with no cognitive impairment. The differences make the intervention very unique and challenging. The similarities, fortunately, make it doable.

Differences

- When one works with people without dementia on issues of mental health, crisis, or life change, there is often an expectation of improvement and resolution. While PWESD can learn to cope with and adapt to symptoms of dementia, ultimately—at this point—there is no cure for the disease.

- Memory loss and other cognitive impairment compromises insight, which affects the counseling process as well as functioning in daily life.

- Dementia also impacts the counseling relationship, as there are usually challenges in communicating with PWESD, such as word-finding difficulty.

- PWESD have complex needs as they face ongoing loss of abilities with disease progression.

- While psychotherapeutic techniques will be used, the model calls for more than just talking. The framework blends emotional support with problem-solving, care coordination, and a number of other interventions depending upon each PWESD's situation.

- A structure for counseling becomes more important, to help both PWESD and counselors navigate their sessions together.

Similarities

- As a counselor you are likely to be familiar with such skills as active listening and expressing empathy. These and any other clinical activities you can think of are as relevant to working with PWESD as with anyone else.

- Likewise, roles a counselor plays such as facilitating change or providing education are already likely to be natural to you.

- At its core, counseling can be an elixir of calm and clarity that comes amidst chaos. The counselor's receptivity offers a potential doorway through turmoil to restored equilibrium. While progressive dementia requires continual recalibration, the PWESD follows the same path as other clients from the exile of solitary struggle to the relief of more buoyant coping ability.

These commonalities with any therapeutic venture can give you confidence in working with PWESD. While it is normal to feel some apprehension before proceeding into this terrain, you may also be curious and excited! Combining the art of your own counseling style with the science of technique you will learn here should provide you with an excellent foundation for doing this work. And, as with anything else, we all learn as we go along. If you have done support groups with PWESD then this individual approach is likely to resonate with you quickly and easily. If you haven't done groups but have the appropriate qualifications, I invite you to begin the journey with a trust in your existing skills and intuition, a sense of openness to what you will discover, and a willingness to be taught and guided by those PWESD with whom you work.

Accentuate the Positive

You might be heartened to know that, while this approach addresses grief, uncertainty, and many other difficulties that come with having dementia, it also focuses on the resilience and wellness that remain. We will explore crafting the paradox of simultaneously facing deficits while also building upon strengths. People are more likely to be depressed and angry without help finding their potential to pre-vail than with it, and often flourish when reoriented to this possibility.

A Word about Families

Much has been written over the years about caregiving and even about counsel-ing family members. This book focuses primarily on counseling PWESD because it hasn't been as prominently addressed. The early stage of dementia is the unique time when diagnosed individuals and their families have the gift of ability to work together. In fact, the term "care partners" used from here on was originally coined by PWESD who felt that it reflects less of a sense of burden and more of a team approach. In the pilot project described in Chapter 13 (which had short, one-time funding) counseling was designed for PWESD with families involved to a limited extent. Ideally, counseling should be widely available to both PWESD and care partners, both separately and together, to maximize effective coping with the disease.

You will read more about family issues and relationships when we walk through the framework, and then in Chapter 7.

Purpose and Benefits of the Program

We begin this journey, then, looking at the palette of potential goals and positive outcomes that can result from counseling with PWESD.

Purpose

Here is the canvas:

- Support in facing the diagnosis of early dementia
- Information to understand the illness
- An opportunity to talk and work through issues that is usually not available elsewhere
- A relationship with a clinician who listens with attention, kindness, and respect
- A focus on competence rather than only disabilities
- Improved coping ability—using the framework of Emotional Adjustment, Practical Coping Strategies, and Lifestyle Issues

Benefits

Here is what we hope the painting will look like:

Benefits to PWESD

- Increased well-being and acceptance from understanding and acknowledging the illness

- Improved self-esteem and mood from working through feelings

- Increased capacity to manage daily symptoms and challenges that accompany the illness

- Knowledge of good self-care skills

- Adaptations to changes in abilities and lifestyle

- Education about the disease, research, available medications, programs, and resources

- Decreased isolation

- Connection with the dementia service system before times of crisis

- A sense of going on with life, and having the best one possible

Benefits to Families

As explained, while families are not a central part of the program as it is written here, having PWESD in counseling can prepare them for better communication and interactions with relatives. Family members can be invited into sessions to talk about issues that have come up. Counseling discussions may enable PWESD to participate with their care partners in the following areas:

- Emotional catharsis

- Problem-solving around needed adjustments at home

- Decisions about important future legal, financial, health, and care planning

Staff/Agency Benefits

Counselors (and if applicable, their agency settings) can receive the following benefits:

- "State-of-the-art" skills in counseling this population

- Enhanced capacity to provide specialized care

- Leadership in a needed area of the field

- Rewarding enrichment through both personal growth and professional development

- Increased morale and job satisfaction, which are critical in this intense and difficult field

- More points of entry/engagement for PWESD into the dementia continuum of care

- PWESD and families learning about and attending other agency programs
- Expanded network of mutual referrals through increased community awareness and collaboration

In Terms of Terminology

Since a variety of terms are routinely used when referencing early-stage AD and some have recently changed, a quick review is offered here. However, while a solid understanding of AD and related disorders is most important for a counselor to have, this basic information is beyond the scope of this book. It is readily available through such excellent organizations as the Alzheimer's Association, Alzheimer's Foundation of America, and Alzheimer's Disease Education and Referral Center.

Definitions

Alzheimer's disease versus dementia versus other disorders—"Dementia" refers to symptoms that affect a person's daily life functioning, including difficulties in memory, thinking, and behavior. Dementia can be caused by many different conditions. Some are reversible, such as depression, malnutrition, or medication reactions. AD is the most common form of irreversible dementia. Others include vascular (stroke-related) dementia; Lewy body dementia (which causes Parkinson-like physical symptoms); and frontotemporal dementia, which can affect personality, behavior, and language.

Getting an accurate diagnosis is of paramount importance. A thorough, multidisciplinary evaluation conducted by specialists in geriatrics and memory disorders can rule out and attend to any treatable causes of symptoms. This will include a medical examination and history; blood tests and brain imaging; and tests of memory and cognition (e.g., word-finding or judgment).

This book is focusing on dementia due to Alzheimer's or other progressive disorders. Within this broad spectrum the features vary depending on the portion of the brain affected. Therefore, each person has to be assessed individually to see whether insight, emotional acuity, and communication skills are intact enough to enable the person's participation in counseling.

Early-stage—Until quite recently, clinicians and researchers used the terms "early-," "middle-," and "late-stage" Alzheimer's disease to describe approximate points in the progression of the disease course. The increasing degree of impairment over time was correspondingly categorized as mild, moderate, or severe. Generally, people with *early-stage* Alzheimer's disease are those of any age who have only mild impairment. For example, little assistance is initially needed with self-care activities. Over time, confusion and forgetfulness become apparent as cognitive and functional abilities are increasingly affected by the illness. More things that were easy to remember, learn, or do become challenging. Many individuals in the early stages of Alzheimer's disease are aware of and concerned about these changes, unlike individuals in the later stages, whose capacities for introspection and comprehension are compromised.

There are certain behaviors that care partners must cope with that also tend to correlate to the individual's stage or level of impairment. For instance, repetitive questions and losing one's train of thought are common in the early stage of dementia, while wandering or inability to recognize others indicates more severe impairment. Care partners of PWESD may be newly learning about the disease and the service system, and struggling with such decisions as whether individuals should continue to drive or live alone. As the disease progresses, of course, more care and supervision are required in all areas of daily life. However, the rate of progression varies for each person, and in some cases functioning with minimal decline may plateau for a number of years.

Early dementia—This is another way to refer to the beginning point in the ill-ness, when symptoms of cognitive and functional impairment are relatively mild.

Newly diagnosed—This refers only to the recency of diagnosis, which does not predict the severity of impairment. People seek diagnostic evaluation at varying points in the disease course. Thus, a person's cognitive status is more accurately described by the stage (early, middle, or late) or level of impairment (mild, moderate, or severe) than by the amount of time since diagnosis.

Early onset/younger onset—This refers to a person whose symptoms of dementia began before the age of 65, regardless of their current stage or level of impairment. Younger and older people who have early (mild) dementia have some similar and some different issues because of where they are in the life span. Both are faced with emotional adjustments and disruptions in identity, lifestyle, and relationships. So it is important to determine each person's needs individually rather than make assumptions about the relationship between age and the effect of the illness on life circumstances.

Revised Guidelines

At the time of this writing, new guidelines are being adopted for diagnosing AD. The stages are now characterized as beginning before symptoms are apparent and are based on biological changes in the brain. The three new stages are preclinical, MCI, and Alzheimer's dementia.

Preclinical is a term that currently only applies in a research setting. It is identified by brain imaging that shows nerve damage and levels of protein in the blood and spinal fluid that may indicate the presence of AD. These brain changes can start as much as ten years before symptoms of disrupted memory or thinking occur.

Mild cognitive impairment (MCI) is a stage marked by symptoms of memory and/or other thinking problems that raise concern but don't interfere with one's independence or daily activities. Some people with MCI progress to Alzheimer's dementia, while others don't. They won't know at the time of diagnosis whether this will happen or not.

Alzheimer's dementia is now the final stage of the disease in which symptoms such as memory loss, word-finding difficulty, and impaired reasoning are significant enough to affect a person's ability to function independently.[4]

There is some concern that the new guidelines will cause confusion. People who were previously told that their diagnosis was early AD may now be referred to as MCI; which was previously a stage between "normal" and dementia. Research is focusing on the biological and cognitive changes that lead to worsening problems.[5] But meanwhile, some experts predict that the changed guidelines will result in a two- to threefold increase in the number of people being told they are probably on their way to getting AD.[6] With the third stage now bearing the blanket term "Alzheimer's dementia," one hopes that the hard-won gains in raising awareness, challenging fear and stigma, and distinguishing early dementia as a time of remaining capabilities will not be set back.

Clearly these new guidelines are somewhat controversial, and, again, beyond our scope. But their impact looms large. The reason and hope for them is to develop and test medications earlier so they will be more effective against dementia. Medications currently ease symptoms for some people for some period of time, but they don't work for everyone and are still not able to prevent or cure progressive dementia. Whether or not medication works for a given person, information and support are equally critical.

This brings us back to our focus here, as counseling can help by giving people the opportunity to talk about the illness, understand it, and plan for the future. The terms "early-stage" and "early dementia" (and those early onset who are in the early stage) as described earlier refer to the population that this program targets. Doctors vary in whether and how they are using the new guidelines. Suffice it to say that many of the concepts and practices presented here can also be applied to people diagnosed with MCI.

Overcoming Barriers

The push to recategorize early dementia and diagnose the disease before symptoms even appear makes the need to enhance our current infrastructure even more urgent. There are still a number of hurdles ahead. But if we reach people sooner and offer the chance to deal with their situation, we can impact present quality of life *and* potentially make future transitions between levels of care less traumatic.

One barrier is our gap in services. Even in progressive and service-rich regions, senior centers and other providers may try to deny that memory loss exists in their population. It is imperative to change this climate. Those who are experiencing dementia should feel unashamed and welcome to try to participate rather than being ignored. They can then be respectfully connected with settings that better meet their needs if that is what's most appropriate.

Dementia care agencies also have multiple constraints. Funding is scarce in these economic times, and pressure is on to serve larger numbers of clients with fewer resources. Individual counseling is time and labor intensive. Yet it very directly impacts coping with the disease. This foundation can offset additional (and likely more expensive) problems people may have in the future.

Education and outreach to the general public and to agencies serving seniors are critical. Changing the usual "storyline" from the focus on incapacity challenges widespread misperceptions and stigma. This will be discussed in Chapter 9.

Also, clinicians must be trained so that they are comfortable offering counseling to PWESD. Many in the dementia care field are skilled at helping families manage "problem behaviors" or assessing risk in the mid to late stages. The professional's role in the early stage, though, may more often be one of mediator or negotiator. PWESD's dignity and autonomy must be upheld where possible, and their involvement facilitated. For example, a person who is resisting help may newly need oversight in some areas—but actually also have an overbearing family. We will look at some of these roles and their complexities.

Then there is the factor of the family's discomfort. Even questioning how much the person with dementia should be told presents an obstacle in including them in discussions about their diagnosis. Giving families support and guidance at this beginning point in the process can set a positive tone and style for many future interactions to come. This will be explored further.

Another barrier has been professionals' discomfort in working directly with PWESD. Counselors' feelings and issues are provoked in the normal course of this work. But stereotypes, fear, and uncertainty exacerbate these reactions. Chapter 4 will explore these and other countertransference issues. Learning specific, constructive communication techniques for people with early dementia can also make the idea of counseling less formidable. These will be addressed as well in Chapter 4.

And finally, there is the barrier of the PWESD's resistance. If they are defensive or in denial about their deficits, we may think we shouldn't push them. The delicate issue of denial will be discussed further in Chapters 3 and 6.

Continuing On

The disparate ingredients of this introductory stew create the backdrop for the counseling program. Great progress has been made in the early dementia care field, but there is much new work to do. Working together, perhaps we can take it to the next level.

This publication certainly can't solve all the problems that PWESD and their families have. It can't even tell you how to intervene in every situation you might encounter. But it does give you a manifesto of the special challenges faced by PWESD, strategies to address them, the texture and architecture of the counseling relationship, and a protocol for putting it all together.

CHAPTER 2

A Framework for Coping with Early Dementia

People newly diagnosed with early-stage dementia often report that they are given no guidance about *how* to cope with the distinctive challenges associated with their condition. This early-stage counseling approach operates within a framework that has three domains of coping, which are termed Emotional Adjustment, Practical Coping Strategies, and Lifestyle Issues. Each is independently relevant, while also interrelated with the other two, as shown in Figure 2.1. Generally speaking,

Emotional Adjustment has to do with integrating the psychological impact of having AD;

Practical Coping Strategies involve managing the challenges of everyday functioning; and

Lifestyle Issues have to do with adapting to changes in abilities, activities, roles, and relationships.

The framework provides a structure to assist the counselor in both identifying and addressing the issues that are present in different areas of a person's life. Yet it allows for flexibility and variability in what those issues might be for each individual, and the individual's readiness to deal with them. You will see in Chapter 10 that the model mandates that PWESD who engage in this counseling must be both willing *and* able to work on their many issues. Also, a precondition of using this framework is a relationship of trust between the person and the counselor, which will be discussed in Chapter 4.

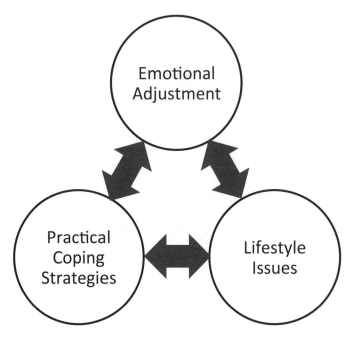

Figure 2.1. Three Domains of Coping with Early Dementia (Copyright © 2011, by Robyn Yale)

Each of the three domains of coping is further illustrated in Figure 2.2 with six elements, which will be detailed more as we move along. The three dimensions of coping may be dealt with either individually or simultaneously. They are intended to be overlapping rather than linear. People may choose or need to focus on one area when they begin counseling, but because the areas are interconnected, it is likely that all three will eventually be incorporated. Each domain is an integral aspect of coping with early dementia; working on one without the others would not be as effective. For example, one person might come in wanting to learn about improving her memory through cognitive exercises, and then once the counseling relationship is established she may become more open to facing the emotional reality of her diagnosis. Another person may have to reach some level of emotional acceptance of his condition before he is able to acknowledge the need for memory aids (or give up driving or designate power of attorney).

Any issue you can think of fits into the framework, as illustrated by these additional examples: Losing the ability to do one's job obviously necessitates lifestyle change—but also has an emotional impact. Grappling with such emotional issues

EMOTIONAL ADJUSTMENT	PRACTICAL COPING STRATEGIES	LIFESTYLE ISSUES
Acceptance of Condition	Stress Management	Social and Vocational Activities
Existential Issues	Memory Aids	Future Planning
Identity	Communication Techniques	Family Relationships
Expressing Feelings	Physical Wellness	Asking For/Accepting Help
Resilience	Cognitive Exercise	Service Utilization
Relating to Others	Support System	Problem Solving: Safety Issues

Figure 2.2. Elements of the Three Domains of Coping with Early Dementia (Copyright © 2011, by Robyn Yale)

as identity and self-esteem caused by having the disease affects how individuals reconfigure their time and activities. The progressive loss of autonomy has to be coped with emotionally (what's it like to need help with things?) as well as on a daily practical basis (e.g., how to remember the day's schedule?) and in terms of lifestyle (can one spend the day alone anymore?). Similarly, whether or not one is facing the reality of the Alzheimer's diagnosis or is in denial can profoundly affect family relationships.

The value of the framework, then, is that it raises awareness in both the counselor and the counselee of the interplay of these three areas of coping. It also provides a blueprint for the intervention, as well as a means to evaluate it. As we proceed, the framework will be presented by explaining the unique challenges faced by PWESD; discussing how to work with these challenges; examining the counseling relationship; and looking at how individualized goals can be set before and reviewed after the counseling sessions.

Upon reflection, you may think of different ways to categorize the components of the framework. For example, stress management could fall under emotional adjustment; or tending to physical wellness can be thought of as a lifestyle issue. There is no right or wrong way to classify them, and a framework is just an artificial construct. In fact, this just underscores the main point that the three domains are inextricably interwoven, and all need to be kept in mind when offering counseling to PWESD. Think of them as portals of access to the dynamic aspects of a person's experience, as illustrated when we put it all together in Figure 2.3, The Framework For Coping With Early Dementia.

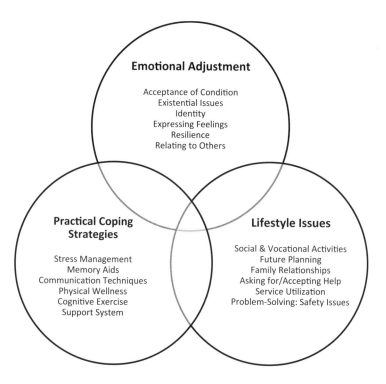

Figure 2.3.   Framework for Coping with Early Dementia (Copyright © 2011, by Robyn Yale)

Identifying the Special Issues and Challenges Facing People with Early-Stage Dementia

Overview

Alzheimer's disease affects each person differently. It progresses at different rates with different symptoms along the way. Despite this individual variability there are many challenges common to those in the early stages. This is the time of the onset of problems, when impairment is substantial yet still relatively mild. At this beginning point, the issues are unique from those experienced in the middle and later stages of the illness.

What follows is a discussion of many issues that arise, categorized into the three domains of the coping framework. Again, keep in mind that this organization is somewhat arbitrary, and also that the three domains are intertwined. As you read you will get a sense of the various connections, and of how the whole will become greater than the sum of its parts.

Also know that the issues below are multidimensional, are presented in no particular order, and are not meant to represent *all* of the difficulties that may occur. Similarly, every person will not necessarily encounter every problem listed here, and each will have different priorities in working on them.

Finally, *please note that this section only talks about challenges and not solutions.* It will be followed by chapters on the counseling relationship and the therapeutic process *before* getting back to how to address the issues explored here, set goals, and review progress. This structure was chosen deliberately to emphasize the importance of a solid counseling dynamic as a precursor to intervention. To hold our place between the current exploration of the early-stage issues and our later look at dealing with them, each one has a goal statement that summarizes it. This will also serve as the thread between our later discussion of addressing the challenges and then evaluating progress toward goals and the counseling experience.

Special Issues and Challenges

Part 1—A Framework for Coping: Emotional Adjustment

People who receive a diagnosis of early dementia typically experience a myriad of overwhelming emotions, and usually have few opportunities to process them. In many interventions and resource materials about coping with dementia, practical issues (e.g., memory aids) and lifestyle issues (e.g., activities) dominate the focus. In this model, the emotional domain of coping pays attention to the equally critical psychological impact of having AD, as shown in Figure 3.1. An explanation of the six elements that encompass it follows.

A. Acceptance of Condition

There are a number of different aspects to whether or not one accepts that one's condition is AD.

Understanding the Disease

People with Alzheimer's have varying degrees of understanding of the disease; awareness about the severity of their own cognitive impairment; and levels of acceptance. They may have many questions, including how to recognize it, whether it might get better, or how fast it will get worse. Some people seek out information about AD and are able to integrate what they learn into various coping strategies.

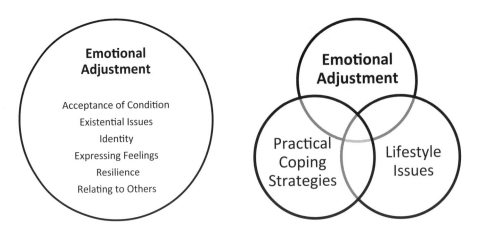

Figure 3.1.   A Framework for Coping: Emotional Adjustment (Copyright © 2011, by Robyn Yale)

Others can do this with support and assistance. But many people do not initiate gaining knowledge about the disease. Often, no one has offered to answer their questions, assuming that they can't understand or handle it or will be too upset. In some cases this may be true. That is why all that follows is based on a thorough screening process to ensure ability and willingness before proceeding with counseling. Too often, though, it's just a matter of people routinely not having the opportunity to ask their questions and get frank answers. Even those capable of insight may remain fearful and isolated without information. While the facts can be traumatizing, knowledge is still power. As with any other illness people are entitled to know—if they want to—what it is, what can or can't be done about it, and how to modify their practices and expectations. Thus, this emotional piece is a springboard that enables us to simultaneously look at the practical and lifestyle implications of the disease.

Acknowledgment of the Condition

Some people are able to admit that they have a diagnosis of AD and that their condition causes certain deficits. Others resist this truth or may fluctuate in their awareness and acceptance. This can be helped or hindered by such factors as whether or not they were even told that their diagnosis was dementia, and how others around them perceive and are dealing with it. Furthermore, how one copes with this involves one's emotional resourcefulness and available support. It may also depend on how one has dealt with other situations in one's life in terms of being open to information and discussion about health or other issues, versus preferring to avoid or simply be private about them. And people may be very reluctant to disclose the diagnosis to others, such as friends or an employer, for fear of the reaction or potential repercussions of doing so.

Acceptance

Understanding the disease and being able to acknowledge one's condition can facilitate coming to terms with it. People have varying levels of openness to doing this, and when we meet them, individuals will be at their own point in the process, working through it at their own pace. Some people don't have the desire or capacity to reach this point, and since they never will they would not be right for this counseling program. Others fluctuate back and forth between admitting that they have the disease or its symptoms and feeling that they don't. And still others are quite able to reach a full degree of acceptance. Because there is such an infinite range of possibilities, we have to meet each person we see with fresh eyes and a bucketful of patience. For example, someone you first meet may not be able to say that she should give up driving. But as the trusting counseling relationship grows she can say that there have been recent times when she got lost while on a familiar neighborhood route. Or someone else may eventually go from insisting that he never misplaces things to admitting that this happens once in awhile. These are small but important steps in the big, scary process of acceptance, and doing it incrementally makes it more possible for some people. Conversely, not having the opportunity to talk through and reach acceptance may leave people more confused because they have no explanation for what they are experiencing. It is more difficult to acknowledge something that isn't fully known—so one reasonable response to that is resistance.

A Special Note About Denial: Denial is a complicated and sensitive issue. Individuals do not always accept the diagnosis or admit their difficulties. When someone denies that symptoms are as severe as they are or questions the validity of the diagnosis, it is important to understand that denial can be multifactorial. Cognitive impairment can affect insight, awareness, and the ability to remember that one has dementia. Denial can also be a defense mechanism against emotional pain. In some people it may be both a neurological and a psychological barrier to seeing the reality of their situation. Furthermore, those who were never told their diagnosis and those who are surrounded by the denial and avoidance of family members and others (such as facility staff) may also less readily acknowledge their condition. And, shame, due to the stigma with which people with dementia are regarded, can keep people from admitting their difficulties. Finally, denial can also be based in fear of loss of control: *if I admit this, you will think I'm incapacitated and start taking over my life.*

Each person works through the difficult process of acceptance differently. Some remain steadfast in denial, and we would not be working with them here. Others may vacillate between denial and acknowledgment or acceptance from time to time when you see them, or steadily over a period of time. Still others can ultimately move beyond denial. One person wrote about his own journey of facing and integrating his decline taking ten years (his "counselor" was a good listener but did not intervene).[1] The point is that, instead of acquiescing to the common belief that all PWESD are in denial, we need to give individuals the time and the chance to work through all their ambivalence and grief.[2] This plus the safe counseling environment and affirming, empathic approach encourages self-disclosure and the therapeutic discussion that can potentially reduce denial.

We will return to addressing these issues later. For now, let's just say that the PWESD's goal for this area of emotional adjustment can be summarized as follows:

> **GOAL:** Understanding, acknowledging, and becoming more accepting of my condition

B. Existential Issues

After a diagnosis of AD, many people feel adrift because they have been offered no emotional outlet and no strategies for coping. They are typically dealing with monumental issues of loss of independence, changes in self-concept, facing disease progression, and contemplating eventual mortality. Some people are more aware than others that AD is a terminal diagnosis. A spiritual crisis can come from realizing that they may, over time, lose even the memory of their own history. One may be seriously facing for the first time the concept of death and what, if anything, comes after it.

Whether individuals deny or accept their condition as already discussed is often strongly rooted in how they make sense of such existential quandaries as

How much more of my life is ahead of me? What will the tenor and texture of that life be like? They may feel reluctant to discuss these issues with family and friends, not wanting to upset others, not knowing how to verbalize their own feelings, or being afraid to confront these issues about the future themselves.

Additionally, dementia causes many changes that compromise self-sufficiency. Tough questions about capacity in major areas like living alone (or even being home alone) usually don't have clear answers at one point in time. Who makes these decisions—and is the person involved in that process? As autonomy is taken away, PWESD can feel devalued and demoralized.

If one has been diagnosed with early-onset dementia, these issues are especially out of sync at this stage of life. But it's also challenging if one is older. Perhaps additional aging-related health or emotional concerns are already affecting independence. This new development compounds the sense of loss and crisis.

At this juncture, people often question what their life has meant, or how they can continue to feel worthwhile and productive. Lifelong roles played at work or home may be shifting, and it may no longer be possible to participate in activities that were always fulfilling. Without these familiar structures and routines, people can feel very lost. Summarizing our counseling goal in this area into something manageable, then, we arrive at this aim:

> **GOAL:** Working toward finding new meaning and purpose in life

C. Identity

The cataclysmic losses and changes that dementia evokes trigger many issues around identity. Stepping away from a career or other long-held positions or talents can make people feel unmoored and unsure of themselves. It is common to feel overshadowed by becoming "someone with Alzheimer's" because of the public perception that AD is identified with mental illness and immediate incapacity.

Core beliefs about one's self-image are challenged. Self-esteem may be profoundly affected by diminishing capabilities, the need to ask for assistance, and the feeling of being marginalized by others.

Confusion and concern are reflected in such questions as, *Who have I been in my life? Who am I now, and who will I become as this disease shifts my sense of myself? What do I have to offer or contribute now?* People may be so shaken that it's hard to even recall and honor past accomplishments. This leads us to the next goal statement:

> **GOAL:** Redefining my identity and feeling good about who I am

D. Expressing Feelings

People experience a myriad of feelings as they face the major trauma of being diagnosed with early dementia. Such emotions as grief, shock, fear, shame, anger, and worry are understandable as they lose control of what they thought their life would be like from here forward. They may become immobilized and not have anyone available who is aware, comfortable, or skilled enough to help them process what they are going through.

Challenges around having memory loss are extremely frustrating. There are obvious concerns in the present as well as anticipatory anxieties about the unknown that lies ahead.

Given the catastrophic nature of all of this, it is likely that no one in their lives has been talking about anything that might still or newly be positive about the situation, even though there are such nuggets that can be uncovered. Thus our goal here encompasses a range of possibilities:

GOAL: Expressing feelings (both positive and negative) about my situation

E. Resilience

There is an immense amount of adjusting to do when one has dementia, both internally and externally. Initial logistics as well as the progressive changes ahead can make the challenges seem insurmountable. Resilience is the ability to recover from and grow through adversity. The predominant view surrounding a PWESD in the family and larger society is often that, since things can't be as they once were, life as one knows it is pretty much over. No one may have framed AD as a condition that the person affected can handle. In the face of so much loss and bleakness, it's difficult to see the potential for healthy adaptations, new satisfactions, or unusual accomplishments. People can be very hard on themselves because they feel so incapable and deflated. Reframing this into a goal statement, we arrive at the following:

GOAL: Having an attitude of being strong and capable

F. Relating to Others

Everything discussed thus far affects and is affected by how one relates to others. Stereotypes and misperceptions of PWESD may cause them to be treated insensitively or more intrusively than necessary. The general stigma about dementia makes people feel ashamed and that it should remain concealed. Without alternative frames of reference, a sense of helplessness may be reinforced as others avoid or condescend to them. Well-intentioned family members may take over things the person can still do without checking out their assumptions. PWESD may not realize that they can learn to communicate their concerns and feelings about this. Here, then, we arrive at our next goal:

GOAL: Letting other people know that I want to be treated with respect

Special Issues and Challenges

Part 2—A Framework for Coping: Practical Coping Strategies

Memory loss and other cognitive changes that accompany dementia pose many challenges to functioning effectively in daily life. The disease can also affect judgment, decision making, and the ability to complete tasks. Keeping in mind the emotional ramifications we just explored, in the practical domain of coping we examine what can either exacerbate or lessen the impact of symptoms, as shown in Figure 3.2. Discussion of the following six elements is meant to give you an overview of the areas in which special issues arise, rather than a detailed analysis.

A. Stress Management

Having impairment in memory and thinking is very disruptive and frustrating. As with other things in life, how one reacts can be the key to coping either dysfunctionally or successfully. Trying to avoid or resist how things are and force one's way through challenges—or getting mad at oneself—are natural reactions but are typically not very helpful. Usually everyone in the PWESD's life thinks that the person's limitations are now inevitable, and little thought is given to how the stress of the situation might be better managed. The home atmosphere and environment may even be contributing to tension around the illness. Things can easily become overwhelming when expectations haven't been altered and people try to do as much as they always did, and in the same ways. Stress can also affect everything that preceded and follows in our discussion, such as by negatively altering mood, cognition, and even physical health. Given the importance of this area, then, our goal here becomes the following:

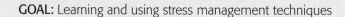

> **GOAL:** Learning and using stress management techniques

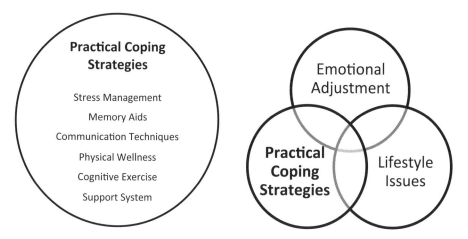

Figure 3.2.   A Framework for Coping: Practical Coping Strategies (Copyright © 2011, by Robyn Yale)

B. Memory Loss

Memory loss is the hallmark of AD, and almost always the first noticeable symptom. It is very distressing to forget appointments or recent events, and to forget what one was going to say or to repeat oneself often. Planning, sequencing, and completing tasks become difficult even with lifelong skills like following a recipe or paying a bill. Losing things and getting disoriented or lost oneself are among the many other ways in which memory loss can impact one's daily life.

Once again, others may assume that nothing can be done, and there may be no one offering guidance on techniques, tools, or reminder systems that can help with these challenges. This leads us to the next goal:

> **GOAL:** Using memory aids and strategies

C. Communication

PWESD may have challenges around communication including word-finding, comprehension, and self-expression. Tracking conversation, keeping focus and attention, and retaining one's train of thought can also become problematic. Some of the non–AD brain disorders may cause additional physical and cognitive difficulties with speech.

The loss of ability to communicate can be very troublesome. It may lead people to withdraw from social situations and other interpersonal interactions. Additionally, when family or friends notice that a PWESD is having a hard time speaking, sometimes they jump in and provide words before the person has time to come up with them. Some people with dementia find this aggravating, while others appreciate help if they are still struggling after a few seconds. This big topic can be summarized with an overarching goal:

> **GOAL:** Enhancing my ability to communicate and informing others about it

D. Physical Wellness

People may not realize the relationship between physical health, mental health, and brain health. Health interventions can't yet be said to prevent onset or progression of AD. But the latest thinking about AD is that what's good for the body is also good for the mind. For example, keeping weight, cholesterol, and blood pressure at healthy levels reduces the risk of other illnesses, which may help to optimize cognitive functioning. Exercise can improve mood as well as blood and oxygen flow to the brain. Dietary, rest, and good sleep habits are also factors in optimal physical (and mental) health.

Wellness interrelates with many other components of the framework, such as cognitive exercise, stress management, and purposeful activity. If PWESD do not practice good self-care or monitor coexisting medical conditions, symptoms of dementia can be exacerbated. Our goal here, then, concerns overall health:

> **GOAL:** Paying more attention to physical exercise, diet, rest, and general health

E. Cognitive Exercise

Cognitive "fitness training" has been an area of intense investigation and differing opinions. It isn't definitively known yet whether this can improve cognitive functioning. But it is believed that the brain benefits from stimulation because connections between brain cells are strengthened. So while activities like memory enhancement exercises may not prevent or cure disease progression, they may contribute to optimal brain health.

People with dementia may assume that they can't perform well in this area. And it will be easier and more appealing for some than for others to practice it. Some may be too discouraged to try, and others may run into problems if they force beyond what is comfortable or attempt things that are past their capabilities. There are a variety of avenues and much that has been developed to offer PWESD. But many people aren't presented with appropriate guidance or opportunities that can help them explore and be successful in this area. This brings us to our next goal:

> **GOAL:** Doing memory and other cognitive exercise activities

F. Support System

It is very easy to become isolated when one has dementia. Friends often withdraw, and the person may not feel comfortable with previous social circles and activities. Some have family members intensely involved with them, but others have little family or relatives that are far away. We've talked about the many feelings that can accompany a diagnosis of dementia, the lack of understanding by others, and the limited availability of counseling services for the person with the disease. So, it is likely that PWESD do not have outlets for talking about all the emotions and changes they are experiencing. This brings us to a critical goal:

> **GOAL:** Getting emotional support from others

Special Issues and Challenges

Part 3—A Framework for Coping: Lifestyle Issues

Lifestyle issues may include changes in activities, abilities, roles, and relationships in work, family, and many other key areas of life. Navigating the present situation as well as thinking about the future—while keeping in mind the emotional and

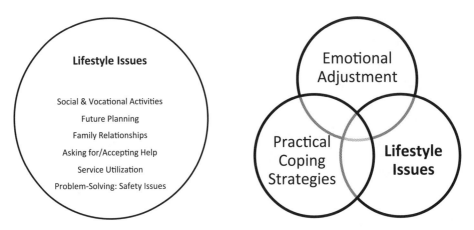

Figure 3.3. A Framework for Coping: Lifestyle Issues (Copyright © 2011, by Robyn Yale)

practical ramifications already discussed—are all tasks here. Helping the person identify these issues as well as accept and adjust to them is the huge challenge in this area of the framework. The lifestyle domain of coping is illustrated in Figure 3.3 and in the following discussion.

A. Social and Vocational Activities

This large area encompasses recreational and work-related activities. Whether currently or more so as time goes along, people become less able to function as they used to in many areas of life. There may be difficulties with favorite or long-standing hobbies. For example, someone who has always been an avid reader might now have trouble focusing or remembering the storyline of a novel. A person with a volunteer role in a social club may find it impossible to keep the books or chair a meeting any longer. PWESD often withdraw from activities because the change in abilities causes stress and shame. Social isolation then compounds fear and poor self-esteem.

Some people with mild dementia can continue working in their job or career successfully for some time, depending on the region of the brain that is required for it. A workplace may be willing to provide help with checking work, or ways to facilitate a person's continuing to offer expertise. Other workplaces don't, and making errors and other consequences of cognitive impairment are cause for losing one's job. When this happens, there can be a profound sense of despair and grief, particularly for those who felt their job strongly defined them. The abrupt change in daily routine, identity, perceived status, and financial circumstances can be extremely difficult to deal with.

In both social and vocational settings, there is also the dilemma of whether, how, and when to tell others about one's diagnosis of dementia. And as we have seen in so many areas of the framework, there is often no one to help PWESD work through these challenging situations and reframe them in a positive way. This leads us to the following goal:

> **GOAL:** Doing and/or developing new social and vocational activities

B. Future Planning

The multitude of changes in capabilities and roles can be extremely tumultuous for a person with early dementia. As we've said, we seek the delicate balance between accepting what's lost and finding new ways to go on with life. At the same time, part of coming to terms with the illness is recognizing that plans must be put in place for the time when impairment progresses further. Dealing with end-of-life issues is something most of us can find overwhelming and would prefer to avoid. It is particularly daunting when compounded by the emotional impact of being diagnosed with dementia, and all the practical challenges of daily life.

Future planning refers here to wills, trusts, powers of attorney, and other matters related to the disposition of assets upon one's incapacity or death. It also concerns advanced health care directives and the anticipation of additional needs for services and a supported living situation. Most of this can only be discussed and designated while one still has capacity. With the uncertainty about the rate of disease progression, the sooner these affairs are settled, the better.

Ending a job due to the symptoms of Alzheimer's disease can be financially devastating. The loss of income and insurance has repercussions immediately as well as for the rest of one's life. There are many financial issues to consider, for example, How will the cost of in-home or residential (and other) care be covered if and when that becomes necessary? Additionally, for those who have always assessed and managed the household finances, when will they no longer be able to do so? To whom will that responsibility go? And there are a myriad of other considerations.

Given the critical and complex nature of this area of the framework, we reach our next goal:

> **GOAL:** Talking about and making future legal, financial, health, and care-
> planning decisions

C. Family Relationships

The three domains of coping apply to family care partners as well as to people with dementia. Family members have emotional reactions, daily practical challenges, and larger lifestyle issues to grapple with. Chapter 7 will discuss this more, and talk about the role of the family in the counseling program.

Roles and relationships within families are inevitably affected by a diagnosis of dementia. For instance, the person may have been the "breadwinner" or the one who took care of the bills; or may have always been seen as "the strong one." Adult children become confused and conflicted as parental boundaries shift. Here again we see the overlap with other parts of the framework. As one of many examples, self-esteem is affected when a person feels disempowered or unsure about this new change in identity.

Families deal with these matters in very different ways. They may be open in discussing them; they may not know how to broach the subject; or they may avoid it entirely for fear of upsetting the person. And, PWESD may handle things in any of these various ways as well. Navigating these dynamics can be very difficult for the person and the family, especially if they don't have a history of open communication.

Families may under- or overestimate the PWESD's present capabilities, resulting in strained interactions and unnecessary intrusiveness. Of course, PWESD may also have unrealistic expectations about what they are able to do, which is stressful for family members. Both sides can feel resentful and come to an impasse.

Many other areas are also relevant here, including intimacy between partners; potential changes in living arrangements; and concerns about the future. How a particular family finds its way through these perplexing issues depends in part upon long-standing dynamics between members and their problem-solving resources.

Much has been written about "caregiver burden." Professionals may not realize that PWESD are often aware of and concerned about how their condition impacts the well-being of their relatives. Families may not be skilled in relating emotionally to PWESD about their condition to facilitate working through the morass of changing circumstances. The joys and aspects of family life that can be celebrated and positively cultivated are often overlooked at this time of crisis and challenge. This leads us to another vital goal:

> **GOAL:** Acknowledging and working on challenges and changes with my family

D. Asking for/Accepting Help

Cognitive impairment makes tasks that were never considered complex—for example, making change at the store—more difficult to do. With changes in routine and so much more in flux, PWESD may now need assistance with such things as remembering appointments or medications, or with shopping or transportation. The extent to which they are willing to seek and utilize help depends in part on overall acceptance of their condition. Since this process for some is a gradual one, coming to terms with needing help may be a step along the way. Friends, family, and professionals can facilitate the types of adaptations we've been discussing to optimize functioning and fulfillment. But the person may be ashamed or afraid of giving up control or becoming dependent. Intertwined with many other areas of the framework, then, we have this delicate goal:

> **GOAL:** Asking for and accepting help from others

E. Service Utilization

PWESD who are isolated and not linked to any dementia care agencies may not know that many now have specialized early-stage services. (It is a problem that some regions still don't, and more work needs to be done to make these services more available.) Even if PWESD are aware of what's out there, they may be fearful of identifying with or trying out these resources. Yet, the continuum of changes ahead as symptoms progress will proceed most smoothly if people do connect with the continuum of care as early as possible. Each person has different interests so no one program can meet everyone's needs. Amidst the flurry of decisions and arrangements involved in adjusting to life with dementia, the person or family has to reach out or be referred to find out about services. Hopefully, they don't fall through the cracks or too strongly resist the idea of resources they may enjoy and find helpful. This, then, brings us to our next goal:

> **GOAL:** Using early-stage support services

F. Problem-Solving: Safety Issues

This far-reaching component of the framework covers a number of general as well as very specific concerns. Driving, managing finances, being home alone, cooking, and medications are among the safety issues even in the early stages of dementia. Note that the title incorporates a constructive approach, emphasizing active participation by the PWESD. Often, though, these are huge areas of worry and conflict that may not be resolved openly within the family.

The most common—and usually the most emotionally charged—safety issue is driving. Driving ability needs to be monitored and periodically evaluated, as the time to limit or stop it is different for each person. Confusion, delayed reaction time, getting lost, impaired visual-spatial perception, and difficulty with multitasking all increase the risk of having an accident. The decision that driving must cease is even more difficult when the person denies having a significant level of impairment. Families are in a tough position with valid anxieties. Yet, driving represents freedom and independence for most people, so taking away the keys is a huge loss to face.

Managing finances is here considered a safety issue in the sense that PWESD can become vulnerable to exploitation through direct mail solicitations, computer and telephone scams, and strangers. Keeping track of accounts and investments, handling money, and paying bills are routine tasks that eventually become compromised when one has dementia. Taking away these and similar responsibilities can be perceived as a grave affront to a PWESD's autonomy, and may be strongly resisted.

PWESD being home alone brings up a host of safety issues. Cooking may become dangerous if people forget that a pot is on the stove, or forget how to properly prepare food. They may lose track of whether they have eaten, as well as whether they have taken their medications or not. On the other hand, going out alone can also be problematic as it's possible to become disoriented and lost. These and other safety-related matters require attention to the final, essential goal:

> **GOAL:** Taking steps to problem-solve safety issues such as driving or managing finances

Special Issues and Challenges: Summary

Hopefully by now, you have a good grasp of the holographic 18-point Framework for Coping with Early Dementia. The three domains of Emotional Adjustment, Practical Coping Strategies, and Lifestyle Issues overlap with and inform one another. What has been conceptualized in this chapter is not intended to be an extensive primer on working with every issue facing PWESD. Rather, the intent was to introduce (or remind) you of the depth and breadth of the journey, which each person experiences differently. From this, you can be mindful of and organize the wide range of challenges and feelings discussed in a way that is useful, pragmatic, and easy to understand. And you can think about where you may need more information and resources to assist in certain areas—to supplement your counseling prowess.

If there is an issue you think of that's not mentioned, it should fit into the framework somewhere—or everywhere. Also bear in mind the ongoing nature of transitions. For example, some may come to terms with needing to retire from a job and find a new way to spend their time, and later come up against not being able to drive there. Furthermore, the domains exist whether or not someone chooses to deal with them. So a person who is resisting help may be angry although not articulating it; or those who don't want to designate powers of attorney may be affected by decisions their family is making without them.

Please keep the framework and its three-dimensional aspects in mind as we go elsewhere before we come back to it. Let them simmer as we prepare the next ingredients, which include the counseling process and relationship. If you'd like to you could meet me at Chapter 6 if you prefer to read about addressing the challenges right after absorbing them. But I'm keeping them distinct purposely, because I believe that first we have to know how to be present with PWESD before we set about intervening with them.

CHAPTER 4

The Counseling Approach and Relationship

The Craft of Counseling

Now that we've explored the many challenges PWESD face, our tale turns us to the fascinating features of the therapeutic landscape. Its terrain is varied, because each person with dementia has a different story—and so does each counselor. Both come to each encounter at a unique point on the life journey, with different perspectives and experiences to make sense of it. Their work together, then, entails both a high level of skill and the lowest common denominator of human searching and exchange.

As we've seen, all PWESD face the reality of having dementia at their own pace—if they do at all. It's impossible to generically prescribe the conduct of counseling sessions. Your intervention will vary every time depending upon the sequelae of the disease and many other factors. It is the relationship itself that provides an anchor in the stormy sea, catalyzing the processes of "coming to terms" and taking action. Our composure and commitment exquisitely model the calm that is possible during this crisis. Persevering through the quest to gain insight, PWESD open to moments of grace and transcendence. With the gentle weapon of self-awareness come the victories of discovery and self-knowledge so crucial to the struggles ahead.

The craft of counseling is a healing art as well as a science. The art is more ineffable. Chiseling away according to the shape of our intuition, the contours of direction to follow emerge. Our sacred attention, kind nurturing, and subtle guidance encourage PWESD to progress on the faith we demonstrate in ability and possibility.

The science includes our words and techniques. It also hinges on the framework described, with its empirical base. The three domains of coping provide a template that is firm yet pliable. This accommodates the complexity of individual variability.

We saw that the counselor will be called upon to play a variety of roles beyond talking about issues of personal growth (e.g., suggesting memory aids or discussing legal planning options). So the approach is not grounded solely in psychodynamic psychotherapy, which examines the impact of long-standing conflicts on one's life. Operating more holistically, we assess the range of the current situation. The elements of our practice are more eclectic.

Your own understanding, skills, and confidence are sure to increase as you proceed to work with PWESD. To arm you for beginning, we'll look now at the theoretical foundation of the model and the dynamic nature of the counseling relationship. We'll also explore who does it, where it goes, and when it ends.

Counselors' Credentials and Preparation

On a very basic level, one aim of this new work is to encourage anyone in relationships with PWESD to become familiar with their issues and interact authentically with them. Everyone from home health aides to nursing home administrators may be called upon to converse directly about a person's emotional experience with having AD. Hopefully these matters are illuminated here in a way that is useful from many different everyday vantage points.

For those who would like to dive into the counseling role, there are very specific requirements. The highly specialized and sensitive nature of the intervention mandates that practitioners have solid credentials, adequate experience, and relevant personal attributes. A background in mental health is essential, but equally important are skills in working with people with dementia and their families.

Ideally, counselors should be licensed. Licenses vary by state but include clinical social workers, marriage and family therapists, and psychologists. Alternatively, a combination of education and equivalent experience is recommended. A master's degree in counseling, social work, gerontology, or a related field plus at least three years in the dementia care field may suffice for someone who is also appropriately trained and supervised.

When early-stage support groups for PWESD were first developed, there was concern about who should facilitate them. As with those groups, this counseling is not traditional psychotherapy. It is a blend of emotional support, education, and practical assistance. It uses a variety of problem-solving and therapeutic techniques. Then, as now, it was clear that many dementia care agencies have non-licensed staff with excellent knowledge and skills—including counseling family caregivers. Knowing relevant resources and referral mechanisms is also critical, as are assessing people and connecting them with services. Personal qualities such as patience, kindness, and active listening abilities help to create the trust so key to talking with PWESD about their lives. So, while a license is preferable, non-licensed professionals who meet the other recommended qualifications can be considered.[1]

The availability of staff to be in a counseling role often determines who can provide the service. Some agencies will have to seek outside practitioners since existing jobs are already demanding. Reimbursement by Medicare and private insurance depends upon licensing, but fees and grants are other sources of revenue. The pool of possible partners includes therapists in private practice, mental health clinicians, geriatric care managers, diagnostic center staff, and those in area agencies on aging. While the counseling service is a lot to develop and maintain, it dovetails with and should be part of the continuum of services available to PWESD and their families in many different settings.

Formal training and experience in counseling are important. Counselors in any field offer consultation, facilitate change, and empower people to achieve their goals. But even well-credentialed counselors without dementia experience will not be well versed in the unique emotional, practical, and lifestyle challenges facing PWESD. Nor will they know how to navigate the communication and other impairments inherent in working with this population. Specialized education will prepare for and increase satisfaction and effectiveness in this role. The Alzheimer's Association, Alzheimer's Foundation of America and similar organizations offer courses on overviews of the illness and the many related psychosocial and care planning issues.

Training must be provided even to those in the aging and dementia fields who have experience with AD in general but not with the early stages. More will then be needed to ensure that this particular counseling approach is conducted in a consistent and constructive manner. Training allows for the discussion of clinical and administrative guidelines, anticipation of unfamiliar situations, and working through any concerns.

For example, there are specific protocols developed to screen and assess potential counselees (see Chapter 10). Trainees can sit in on these interviews to practice the delicate art of talking one to one with people about their diagnosis of AD. Role-plays are another way to simulate interactions in screening and counseling sessions, and an example is provided. Any agency personnel who will encounter PWESD (including those who answer the phone or do intakes) and any related to the effort (such as evaluators for a research project) will benefit from participating in this orientation. Training needs to be provided by individuals with experience in conducting counseling with PWESD.

Following orientation and training, nonlicensed counselors should be monitored and receive clinical supervision from licensed professionals. Peer consultation with qualified colleagues doing similar work can also be helpful for anyone taking this on. Such outside expertise will be invaluable in assisting new counselors to debrief, refine skills, and deal with any of their own issues and feelings that arise in doing this demanding—yet rewarding—work.

Theoretical Foundation: Practice, Research, and Policy

The theoretical underpinnings of this work derive from multiple streams. Within and across the realms of practice, research, and policy lies a vast treasure trove of useful data. An exhaustive review of all relevant literature is beyond our focus. But we can mine a frame of reference to point the way as we move on toward intervention.

Practice

There are, of course, many styles and approaches to counseling. The model detailed in this book is based on some tenets of existential, humanistic, and person-centered therapy. It also builds upon the historical experiences of those in the early dementia field.

From existential therapy we draw the emphasis on confronting profound and fundamental concerns of existence, such as the inevitability of death and the need to find meaning in life despite the suffering that is inherent in the human experience.[2]

Humanistic therapy encompasses a range of life-affirming values like integrity, self-respect, and the potential we have to develop new skills that can enhance our lives. Positive psychology suggests that well-being is more than happiness, as it includes such elements as accomplishment of something worthwhile and engagement in tasks.[3] The relatively recent blending of Eastern philosophy with Western psychology has catalyzed useful practices like mindfulness, which call for presence, awareness, and compassion.[4] The humanistic school is also concerned with responsibility for social change, in the sense of developing organizational and institutional environments in which people can flourish.[5] This fits with our focus on revolution and evolution, in terms of efforts and services that destigmatize dementia.

The person-centered therapy model overlaps with humanistic thought. It emphasizes the assets that people bring with them to deal constructively with and overcome obstacles. The counselor is called upon to use empathy, warmth, and unconditional positive regard as the basic but mighty tools of the change process.[6] Applied to PWESD, we value each individual's worth and dignity as we examine his or her unique experience. We solicit every client's involvement and perspective, respecting personhood and reinforcing strengths.[7]

The early dementia "movement" grew out of this interpersonal dimension of the helping profession. Those conducting early-stage support groups with PWESD found that the intervention decreases feelings of isolation, facilitates grief work, and provides for the exchange of needed information and resources.[8] The curative factors of group psychotherapy, including catharsis and instillation of hope,[9] were found to fit beautifully here.[10] The belief that a therapeutic process is possible with people with dementia had been modestly advocated.[11] Others began to bolster it, finding that when we look beyond stereotypes to understand PWESD's reactions to what they are going through, we can engage with them and enhance their sense of self-esteem.[12] And, feeling valued, PWESD are often willing to self-disclose.[13] Professionals who learn how to relate to PWESD in this deep way find it very rewarding, and improve their competency.[14]

There are now many examples of PWESD writing about what it's like to have dementia. Finding the power to understand and cope with the experience through intense self-reflection is an ongoing, nonlinear process that can occur over many years.[15] They've told professionals and one another what is helpful to them[16] and have become spokespersons to the field and the general public.[17] They've even provided expertise on how the setting and techniques used can make it easier for PWESD to be interviewed for research purposes.[18,19]

Research

Research has substantiated the clinical findings that PWESD can change their coping behavior after intervention. The opportunity to address feelings and concerns in early-stage specific services like support groups helps them accept and adjust to their condition.[20] Listening and processing experience through such psychotherapeutically based work may improve mood.[21] People operate along a continuum of ability to confront and integrate changes in their lives due to the disease.[22] There are a range of responses, and professionals can help PWESD identify and enhance the most effective ones.[23] Despite the difficult feelings that lead to withdrawing from others and activities, attempts are made to preserve a sense of self and to re-create meaning and identity.[24]

Research has been attempting to demonstrate that cognitive fitness programs, social activity, and physical wellness can all impact brain health. Engaging families with PWESD in education can increase coping and health behaviors like improving diet and exercise.[25] Studies have shown that PWESD can articulate preferences and decisions with their families (separately and together) about health care and financial planning matters, trying memory medications, discussing the illness with family and friends, and stopping driving.[26] A cognitive rehabilitation study showing that individualized goals improved performance in such areas as practical aids and stress management[27] was the inspiration for the evaluation tool described in Chapter 13.

There are methodological issues when one is doing research with this population. A carefully constructed and standardized way of interviewing PWESD is essential.[28] The dearth of valid and reliable outcome measures and concerns about randomization into comparison groups are among other important considerations.[29]

Policy

The need for more psychosocial intervention research with PWESD is now heartily recognized. A worldwide network of scientists recently proclaimed that non-pharmacological treatments can improve well-being of those with dementia and their families, and these need to be more widely available.[30] A European collaboration of researchers advocates for the sharing of information between countries about efforts to improve psychological and social functioning, interpersonal relationships, daily activities, and living skills of PWESD.[31]

A current review of 102 qualitative studies covering 3,095 participants across continents found that, while the significant impact of dementia includes conflicts between PWESD and their care partners, they can continue working together to accept and incorporate it into their lives with support over time.[32] Alzheimer's Disease International concurs that, when people are well-prepared and supported, initial shock, anger, and grief are balanced by a sense of reassurance and empowerment. This consortium of national organizations specifically identifies studies on support around reactions to the dementia diagnosis[33] and ways to counteract the effects of stigma[34] as primary goals. And, leading us back to our aim here, the new U.S. National Plan to Address Alzheimer's Disease has among its strategies educating health care providers about education and support resources for people with the disease and their families.[35]

The Potent Counseling Relationship

In counseling people with early-stage Alzheimer's disease, the interaction between the counselor and the individual is of primary importance. In fact, a current synthesis of literature about counseling reaffirms that the relationship matters more to the success of the intervention than which theoretical model or method is used.[36] And we have already come to understand that the context of our approach operates beyond diagnosis to treating the whole person.

Thus, we begin the therapeutic process by building a solid alliance. Positive rapport is the basis for teaching PWESD that, while they can't change or cure their condition, they can learn to live with it. The alchemy of inner transformation is triggered by the counselor's willingness to tolerate their strong emotions and uncertainties. This models the belief that acceptance can be more constructive than resistance.

The work we are doing with PWESD entails some universal issues that we all grapple with. We will be touched, and we can share our authentic reactions as appropriate. There is a genuine reciprocity to the counseling relationship in the way that the counselor uses his or her own self to give support and feedback.[37] The rewards of the counseling don't happen only for the client. We receive and learn from PWESD as well as teaching them.

Some of this is fundamental to any counseling setting. We all want to be heard and treated with respect, and we tend to thrive more when we are. And, as counselors, we are thrilled when our clients achieve personal growth through our efforts. It is especially gratifying with PWESD, though—who have been most often devalued and demeaned.

Creating the Connection

The first step is always to create an atmosphere of comfort and safety. Your kind, dedicated attention fosters trust, which is key to successful clinical conversations.

The use of careful listening, empathic understanding, and complete acceptance will help to cultivate this sacred bond.

Listening

People with dementia feel a loss of control in many aspects of their lives. They may have been embarrassed or otherwise reluctant to share about their condition with others. Or, they may have had no opportunity to do so. Being able to express very personal thoughts and feelings in a safe, confidential setting can help people regain some sense of control, which itself is therapeutic.

Most counselors are trained in active listening. But the road map of our sessions with PWESD is rather new and somewhat nebulous. We also have to trust. Valuing the listening process, we don't rush to fix anything or set an agenda. We are joining them in the journey to make sense of all they are facing. Responding with sensitivity first rather than advice demonstrates to PWESD that we—as well as they—can allow the experience of just being present with feelings, no matter how intense they may be.

Empathic Understanding

One of the counselor's main tasks is to accurately understand the person's feelings and experiences, and to reflect that understanding in a caring manner. PWESD are often acutely aware that other people in their lives are not educated enough about the disease to know what it is like for them. It can be a great relief to engage with someone who is knowledgeable. Conveying sympathy and compassion, we also teach the skill of turning this tenderness toward oneself.

Empathic understanding helps develop a basis for using the technique of reframing as counseling progresses. For example, if the person feels the counselor truly comprehends what it was like to lose her job, she may later better accept the suggestion that it's an opportunity to pursue new interests, like painting or volunteering.

Acceptance

PWESD coming into the counseling relationship may be newly diagnosed, or a period of time may have passed since the diagnosis. They are in varying stages of understanding and adjusting to it on many levels. It is the counselor's job to meet individuals wherever they are in this process. Validating their personhood, inner worth, and existing strengths while also acknowledging the disease is empowering. So much emphasis is usually put instead on their impairments and limitations. The counselor's gentle ferocity in the face of so much fear and trauma is soothing, and extends hope.

Summary

The positive regard common to all counseling encounters becomes even more significant in working with people with early dementia. Engaging in a warm and nonthreatening manner provides an experience unlike what is usually happening in the rest of the person's life. It also offers an alternative and valuable new perspective.

We can always fall back on these most basic principles. At times, we may not be sure how to help. PWESD show us what they need, and the way forward can often be found by staying in the present moment. This bolts the stability and stamina of the counseling relationship to its foundation.

Counseling Dynamics

Working with PWESD can test the mettle of our familiar counseling methods. Chapter 6 will address the specific issues identified in the coping framework in the context of how they impact PWESD. The following section discusses some of these more as special features of the counseling relationship, and provides ideas for maneuvering through them.

More about Awareness and Denial

Denial of cognitive impairment may surface from the first point of contact with PWESD and throughout counseling sessions. You will see in Chapter 10 that the criteria and process for selecting appropriate counselees require that PWESD acknowledge at least some concern about their condition. Additionally, they must be willing and able to talk about it, and interested in doing so. That section in Chapter 10 will outline some ways to approach and engage people that are intended to also be helpful for noncounseling staff who are handling telephone inquiries. Chapters 3 and 6 explain more about how the counselor encounters denial and the factors involved in it.

Now we just want to underscore the tricky nature of denial and how challenging working with it can be. PWESD who are staunch and unwavering in their denial would not have been brought into this counseling situation. If that becomes the case later (even after other techniques are attempted) it would be logical for the intervention to end. You can explain that these individuals don't seem to feel they fit with what you have to offer, and refer them to other resources. But our screening protocol makes this situation highly unlikely.

It is common, though, for denial to fluctuate along a spectrum of resistance and acceptance. After establishing rapport with the counselor, many people are able to make great strides. More information about the illness, more access to their emotions, and the trusted counseling relationship all facilitate working through and coming to terms with the illness for some people. Others, though, can focus on the practical or lifestyle issues without dwelling on—or denying—their emotional experience. Therefore, talking about the illness will be easier with some people than others. Some will more readily articulate their feelings and concerns, others will be more reticent, and then there are many in between who will come to admit their circumstances simply by having the opportunity they never had before to deal with it in this way.

We stay put and reflect what we hear, whether PWESD say they have no problems, many problems, just a few, or "did once." We may hear contradictions within the same conversation or over time. Every person may not get to a place of wholehearted or permanent acceptance. But acting as a rudder, the counselor steers toward the openings. For example, someone may say he doesn't have memory loss, but did recently forget about a date he had set with a friend. If we don't confront or push, but instead ask what that was like and provide support, the person may continue to disclose more about his experiences.

More about Emotional Reactions

It is natural for a tempest of feelings to arise as people get in touch with the enormity of the dementia diagnosis. While not wanting to stereotype, it can be said that some people in this generation of PWESD may be more used to avoiding than confronting inner emotional work through "therapy." We can familiarize them with the process by allowing whatever needs to be expressed, normalizing reactions as understandable and universal, and showing people that there is a way through the sense of being overwhelmed. At the same time, we respect the boundaries of those whose style is not to be emotionally animated.

Depression needs special mention, as it coexists with dementia in many people. Depression can impact the progression from mild cognitive impairment (MCI) to dementia.[38] Depression is an understandable reaction to loss, and can be compounded by such additional factors as biochemistry, social isolation, and other health or life issues. People who have no chance to talk and connect with others may hasten further cognitive decline. Those who become depressed as they face their current reality at least have the potential to be buoyed by support from the counselor and fellow PWESD in early-stage programs—and often are. It is important to have access to psychiatric backup when medication and other mental health expertise are required.

The counselor's composure enables PWESD to desensitize to their fear and learn that they can tolerate their feelings and reactions. Broken open from shattered confidence, our consoling stewards people through catharsis toward restoration. Our therapeutic framework and setting provide a container in which a delicate new chrysalis begins to form.

More about Homeostasis

It is helpful for the counselor to balance the emphasis and tone of the sessions so that they are neither too negatively focused on the upset around having dementia, nor too positively focused on the absence of distress. Rather, both are essential truths: having dementia is very difficult, but people also have remaining abilities. Because we all want equanimity in our lives, there may be a natural fluidity along this continuum; but it is something to which the counselor should stay attuned. For example, answers to questions about memory loss can be given in a straightforward manner, but titrated according to what information is being requested and where individuals are at in their understanding at the time.

The skillful introspection taught through counseling helps those PWESD with insight to seek and maintain some level of homeostasis. Together we acknowledge both sides of the many dualities that are present: the illness and the wellness; the devastation as well as the resilience; the present that occurs before the future. Making room for the grief, we also explore new possibilities. Reorienting people away from dwelling solely on deficits and endings develops a fresh point of view, and an alternate lexicon for the next stage of life.

Counseling Sessions Mirror Outside Life

Memory loss, communication, and fluctuating capacity are examples of ways in which what PWESD experience in their lives are mirrored in the counseling sessions. Since we are screening for people who have the capacity for counseling, these symptoms will be relatively mild. Still, the counselor must learn how to work with them as preparation for effective intervention. They also present chances in "real time" to enable PWESD to understand and handle their symptoms.

Memory Loss

When cognitive impairment shows up in forgetfulness, the counselor can utilize some structural techniques. Review and summarize what's been said. Restate themes and refocus the conversation. Your consistency and patience are reassuring, and also save face. You can explain that memory loss due to AD is exactly what you are here to discuss, and how the two are connected. Point out how what's happening here and now also occurs at home and elsewhere. Ask how they feel when it does, and what they usually do at the time. Demonstrate that there are ways to react to it that can reduce upset about it, in terms of both attitude and management ideas. Write things down with or for them. In this way, we apply the classic focus on the process as well as the content of counseling sessions[39] to our work with PWESD.[40]

Communication

When cognitive impairment shows up in communication deficits, encourage people to try to stay relaxed rather than be overcome with frustration. Our own behavior fosters this if we listen carefully, simplify our language, and allow extra time for responses. We need to be even more comfortable with silence than is usually called for, even though we may be inclined to jump in and take over when people have difficulty finding or understanding words.

Speaking slowly, clearly, and concisely can help people feel more comfortable about conversing with you. Ask specific and direct questions to draw them out, and paraphrase the answers to show they've been heard. You can also look for nonverbal cues to people's affect in their face and body language if they are having trouble expressing themselves. It is always a good idea to ask for permission to assist with speaking, and to check back afterward to make sure that your interpretations are correct. An example would be, "*I think I know what you mean here, is it ok if I give it a try?"* Then follow up with, *"Was I correct that that's what you were trying to say?"*

This will all be a learning experience if you aren't familiar with it. It also teaches PWESD techniques they can share with others in their lives to make communication more successful. And it stays within our ethic of treating the person with respect.

Fluctuating Capacity

When cognitive impairment shows up in fluctuating capacity, know that dementia doesn't present or progress in a straight line. PWESD, like all of us, have good days and bad days. Their moods and abilities may vary some from week to week as well as over the longer term. Aware of this, you can help them to understand it. Attributing symptoms to the disease rather than to inadequacy or lack of intelligence reframes the perception of incapacity. And here again, we teach both our clients and ourselves—in this case—about not having rigid expectations (of either performance or treatment).

Transference and Countertransference

Transference and countertransference are Freudian terms for the dynamic in therapy during which feelings are transferred, or redirected, from one person to another. A detailed analysis is beyond our scope here. But a brief mention reminds us to keep these potential phenomena in mind.

Transference

Transference has to do with PWESD unconsciously reacting to the counselor as though the counselor were someone else in their life. For example, the person may be reminded of her own parent or child, or another family member. For someone with dementia, though, long-term memories are often quite vivid anyway. For our purposes, let's just say that we need to be mindful of the tremendous power of our counseling relationships. Whether stirred by psychological responses or manifestations of cognitive impairment, we revere PWESD's feelings while gently reorienting to the here and now. Reminiscence and therapeutic grief work are among the tools we might use at these times.

Countertransference

Countertransference puts the proverbial shoe on the other foot. The counselor reacts to the person with dementia due to strong feelings and memories about someone else. It may be the counselor's own parent or another family member— perhaps with dementia as well. Counseling professionals are not expected to be immune from these types of psychological responses; in fact they are quite natural and normal. What is important, though, is separating our personal and professional selves. Being aware of and seeking support for our own issues enhances our comfort, functioning, and enjoyment in the counseling role. Clinical supervision, peer consultation with colleagues, and individual therapy can all be helpful with this as well as with processing the emotional demands of working with PWESD.

The Counselor's Role and Responsibilities

Take Care of Yourself

While this work can be very interesting and highly rewarding, it is also intense and stressful. We have to absorb the trauma of others, with all its angst and struggle. We have to tolerate uncertainty about the trajectory of the disease, and of the counseling. Being human rather than perfect, we may be uncomfortable answering difficult questions, not having a cure to offer, or not being able to gauge progress in leaps and bounds. In some cases people may just be taking in the news of their diagnosis and all the changes ahead, not yet ready to act on anything. We need a cornucopia of ways to continually be kind to and replenish ourselves so that we can remain fully present, giving, and receptive.

Define the Limits of Your Role

PWESD have a variety of multifaceted needs, many of which are unmet. Some live alone, or don't have family. Even those who do may be grappling with huge financial, medical, transportation, family, or other issues. They may need to find programs to connect with, or new living situations. We need to be clear—for ourselves and with our counselees—about what we can and can't provide. Being caring and so involved in their lives, this can be quite challenging—especially if no one else is apparent to pick up the slack. We'll have to set limits on phone calls or other time spent outside of sessions to solve the related problems—and then we'll have to stick to the limits set! If we happen to also be care managers and can smoothly integrate more huge tasks into the rest of our jobs, it's ideal. But if that's not the case we'll need to connect with appropriate professionals to get additional services in place.

Know the Community Resources—and Make Sure They Know You

Following from what's just been said, it's critical to be knowledgeable about your local community resources. Case management, family support, medical, mental health, and social services are among those relevant to persons with dementia. You'll also want to be familiar with eligibility and referral protocol as much as possible. Unfortunately, there are often not enough resources in the aging field, and even those available may not have staff trained in working with dementia. More rare still is expertise in early dementia. So, part of laying the groundwork for our own new service is educating professionals in our regional networks about this population, and about what we are doing with them. And then, of course, you must also know and work with the dementia-specific agencies in your area.

Understand and Stay Informed about the Disease

We've covered the need for orientation and training around dementia-related disorders, including the specifics of the early stages. More generally, it's important to keep up with new developments in terms of research and all that's being learned on an ongoing basis. The field is always changing and growing so we need to stay current, and we can share new information with PWESD and their families, too. *Alzheimer's Daily News* and the major dementia care organizations all provide these updates.

Have Protocols in Place

It's wise to have backup consultation available for psychiatric situations that are beyond your expertise. Examples include prescribing medication, working with concurrent conditions (e.g., post-traumatic stress disorder), and dealing with emergencies. Short of this, however, you should know how to assess for risk and intervene around depression and suicidal ideation.

You must also know regulations for reporting suspected elder abuse, neglect, or exploitation. These areas can be incorporated into initial staff training in agency settings.

Be Culturally Sensitive

Depending upon where you live and practice, you may encounter PWESD with diverse cultural backgrounds. While this intervention is potentially helpful to anyone, there may be barriers of which to be aware. Language is one, as are taboos against seeking help outside the family, or disclosing emotion. Beliefs about the meaning of dementia also vary. At the same time, it's important not to stereotype each person within a certain nationality. Asking if there are cultural norms that might be in play allows us to neither overlook nor overgeneralize about the impact of culture on each counseling relationship.

Since some people may not even come forward for the service, we need to incorporate outreach to community leaders, relevant professionals, and media in diverse cultural networks as part of the start-up efforts in our regions.

Terminating Counseling

Since we are examining counseling from many different angles, we'll conclude this section with a look at how and when we end the relationship. Chapter 12 will talk about the administrative aspects of having either a time-limited or an ongoing service. Here we investigate the process of stopping counseling, whether the end point is fixed or variable.

Ideally, counseling should be provided as long as it can be helpful. There may, however, be constraints around how long it can continue such as lack of reimbursement or other funding. The decision to offer a set number of sessions or leave this more open-ended must be made, then, on a case-by-case basis. It will depend upon the setting, the available resources, and the PWESD. In either situation, termination—that is, the ending of the counseling relationship—must be handled gingerly and respectfully by the counselor.

If the service is time limited, a minimum of eight weeks is recommended. In this case, termination is built in—which poses one set of issues. The time frame is very clear, and the process is nonnegotiable. However, there is so little time to work together that counseling may end before the multiple and complex challenges a person is facing can be tackled in depth. As we saw with early-stage support groups, people often don't want to stop once they are connected with support. If they are benefiting from the alliance, they may have renewed feelings of loss and abandonment when this occurs. Yet, it is still possible to have a sense of accomplishment and to manage this situation if that's the way it has to be.

If counseling is not limited to a certain period, the time for termination is determined as each situation proceeds. This poses another set of issues. A long-term relationship allows more time for a person to understand and come to acceptance of the disease before having to give up things or make other difficult changes. In some cases, termination happens naturally. People may reach a sense of completion, or choose to stop; or they may have unforeseen health, family, or other concerns that cause counseling to end.

In other cases, PWESD may reach a point at which they are no longer comfortable or otherwise able to participate. Disease progression can affect such needed abilities as attention span, speech, and comprehension. When this happens, it falls upon the counselor to consider disengagement. Periodic reassessment of whether a person remains aware of and acknowledges the symptoms of dementia and seems to be benefiting from counseling is recommended (if it's not obvious). Communicating your concern as soon as it becomes apparent allows for a period in which the counselor and counselee can agree to reevaluate the situation together before actually terminating the counseling sessions.

Whether counseling is time limited or ongoing, a smooth transition out of it is essential. Let's look closely at the steps involved:

Lay the Groundwork

It is helpful to have a verbal and/or written understanding before you begin about how the number of sessions will be determined. You can then talk about that counseling which is time limited as it proceeds, so that the end doesn't seem to come abruptly. In longer-term relationships, you can alert the person and family if you begin to notice that cognitive decline might interfere. Examples of warning signs include decreased insight, disorientation, or being tangential in conversation. You can explore whether this has been gradual or more sudden, in case it is due to an acute physical illness or emotional upset, or if anything out of the ordinary is happening in the home environment. You can also ask how the person feels about continuing with counseling.

Try for a Mutual Decision

Through this collaborative process you may agree, disagree, or not be sure whether to continue with counseling. If decline was situational it may be temporary and improve. Or, it may not improve. In some cases, it might not seem appropriate to confront the person with your concerns. But more often than not, because you have been working together, it is possible to be gentle but honest. You may agree to monitor things and raise the discussion again a few sessions later. Talking about what it will be like to stop seeing one another and outlining options for what comes next are good preparation for the eventual inevitable. We'll be talking about family in Chapter 7, but keeping them apprised is important here. You can suggest as part of this that they look with the PWESD at some of the local programs that might now be more appropriate for them.

Give the Opportunity to Say Good-bye

This is an essential piece of losing any interpersonal relationship, and since PWESD have already had many losses with more ahead, extra emotional support is in order. Encourage them to share feelings about ending the experience and the impact it has had. Address fears or other concerns.

Acknowledging the ending is always integral to the counseling experience. It provides an opportunity for PWESD to review, summarize, and consolidate gains. It also enables counselors to get feedback on their efforts and the program, learning what was or wasn't helpful. Most importantly, we want PWESD to have the ending of the counseling relationship be as positive as the beginning, so that they still feel valued, and like they can face the future.

Have a Follow-up Plan

Sometimes we can end the counseling relationship but stay connected with the person and family. For example, an Alzheimer's Association chapter or other organization might be able to integrate the PWESD into care consultation or family support that they are already mandated to provide. It will be less intensive and have a different focus, but still offers continuity.

Hopefully the next steps also include connecting the person and family to other community resources. It may now be time for adult day care, or early-stage programs or activities that are more recreationally focused. Ancillary professionals can be engaged for other needs. However, making these linkages is problematic if there are few qualified professionals or relevant programs in your region.

This brings us back to the need for ongoing revolution, and the evolution of additional infrastructure! In the bigger picture, we need to train and partner with others in our communities to get them involved. Things are certainly going to keep happening after we stop seeing these folks in counseling, and who will bear the responsibility? It's recommended that you document the needs for more counseling and follow-up services than you have available, and submit this to your administrators, funders, and policymakers.

This is one of many transitions that are likely to be ahead for PWESD and their families. If we help them handle it effectively, they will learn that successful adjustments are possible as the disease progresses. They can see that they aren't failing, or disappearing—they are just going on to whatever will better meet their needs at that moment. And as counselors, we will feel less distressed ourselves if a good aftercare plan is in place.

Allow Your Own Reaction

The counselor's reaction to termination also needs special attention. Termination is tough. We took this terrible disease by the horns, developed strong bonds, and worked our hearts out. We're concerned about how PWESD and their families will do when they have to leave our purview. If we provided a short, time-limited intervention we may feel we couldn't do enough. If we saw the PWESD declining, we may be upset by it. We have to take care of ourselves as we go along—emotionally, physically, spiritually, and in all practical ways.

We don't have all the answers, and we can't slay the dragon. But we have offered something that was certainly a lot better than nothing. Our oasis of solace and safety set the tone for the journey ahead. The counseling relationship itself authenticated reality while also offering hope and the means to cope with it. Without this, those with whom you worked might have remained uninformed, isolated, and depressed. Even within eight weeks, it's likely that you've done a lot of good beyond what can be measured.

It's a skill to bring closure to the counseling connection. It can be very challenging. But it's also manageable. Please don't let it stop you from engaging in this work, if you are otherwise so inclined.

CHAPTER 5

The Counseling Process, Techniques, and Goals

The Therapeutic Process

Let's now take the next step in our story, which is to link what's been relayed about counseling with the upcoming chapter on addressing the three domains of the coping framework. The means of that linkage is the therapeutic process. Because each person with Alzheimer's is so unlike every other, and because each counselor has his or her own style, this unfolding is intended to be fluid and flexible. Still, it flows externally through a somewhat predictable route.

Our progress with PWESD has several components. One is the counseling relationship that we've been talking about. Another is the immense inner work the PWESD must do. These are both somewhat intangible, yet they make up the engine that drives us down the path. There are also all the coping strategies and changes we'll be covering next. And finally, there is the more mechanical aspect, which has to do with the configuration of our time together.

What's described here begins after the initial screening and intake interviewing has determined appropriateness for counseling (discussed in Chapter 10). So, you will already have some background information. Now you begin to explore further the ecology of the person before you: What are the environments that the person operates in? What are the person's daily habits and patterns? What is the nature of the person's interactions with the people in his or her life? In what ways is having dementia impacting the natural order of things? What resources does the person have, and which resources are needed?

From this comes the formation of a road map. Think of the general course of action that follows as the gears behind the turning of the wheels. Note that they operate synergistically, rather than one at a time. Figure 5.1 provides a graphic representation of the process.

- *Develop a trusting relationship*—Along with the methods previously suggested (e.g., respect and careful listening), it can be helpful to tell the person a bit about your own orientation. S/he is not likely to know that there is an early dementia "movement" (and if you didn't know it before either, you are now part of it!). This usually piques interest and enthusiasm, and from here you can begin to ask about what's brought the person to see you.

- *Determine where the person is in terms of understanding and acknowledging his or her condition*—This will either become apparent in your conversation, or you can attempt to get at it in ways explained elsewhere.

- *Assess impairments as well as strengths*—Hear what the person says—and does not say but you pick up—about speech, memory, and other cognitive deficits.

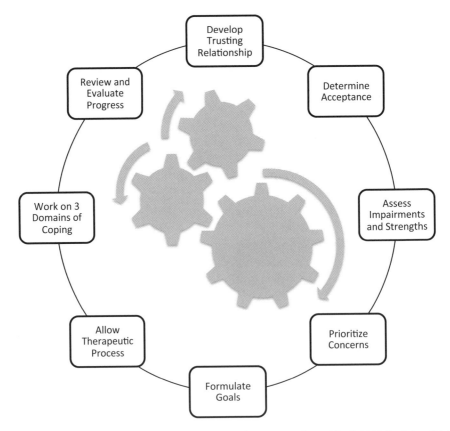

Figure 5.1.   The Early-Stage Alzheimer's Disease Counseling Process (Copyright © 2011, by Robyn Yale)

Listen also for things like what the person is good at or enjoys, or other positive characteristics.

- *Prioritize concerns*—Pay particular attention to red flags, such as the person's living alone, safety issues, or feeling depressed.

- *Formulate goals*—This will be discussed later in this chapter and constitutes your plan for the counseling.

- *Allow the therapeutic process*—As we motor along, however slowly, hopefully the person comes more to terms with his or her situation to at least some extent. The chasm between despair around diagnosis and the ability to move forward with life is seen as one that may be crossed, with your help and new coping strategies.

- *Work on the three domains of coping*—Your goals will guide you to the actions needed to address and integrate the emotional, practical, and lifestyle issues identified.

- *Review and evaluate progress*—See how far you've been able to come together and what needs to happen next. A way to construct this flows from the goals and will be suggested in Chapter 11.

Techniques and Tools

There are a number of ways to supplement the format of the counseling sessions. Here are a few suggestions.

- *Introduce topics*—You can start your meetings by reviewing the previous week's themes and issues. See if a topic emerges from this, or invite the person to say what feels important to discuss. It's good to let the individual initiate topics if possible, but to always have some in mind to bring up if you need them.

- *Provide literature*—You might put together a folder for purposes of orientation, with information about your agency or practice and about the disease. However, choose literature that is not too daunting and is geared toward PWESD. You might also provide a bibliography of books written by and for people with dementia, of which there are now quite a few. Poetry, prose, videos, newsletters, and web sites can all be suggested. You can look at and discuss some of them together. Your local Alzheimer's Association or other organization should have lists of these materials available.

- *Have relevant materials*—You could offer, for example, sample power of attorney forms; or show pillboxes, calendar systems, or other memory aids.

- *Talk about services*—Providing various agency brochures begins to familiarize PWESD and their families with the resources they may need now or as time goes along.

- *Keep a log*—This may be a suggestion that the person do journaling, or it may be a brief note that you compose together at the end of each session to keep track of where you've been and any decisions that were made.

- *Remember the three-dimensional framework*—Keep in mind that any issue you are working on in one area is likely to have repercussions in the other two. For example, talking about memory aids for the daily practical challenges can have emotional reverberations. Doing life review can get some people to a place of readiness to either surrender or tackle something anew, like one of their activities. Rehearsing for a family meeting may open the door to learning more effective communication strategies. These huge challenges are all interwoven, even if we only focus outwardly on one segment at a certain moment.

- *Assign "homework"*—There may be things that it would be helpful to follow up on during the week. Asking permission to involve family with this end of things can increase the chances of getting it done. Whatever it is needs to be small and achievable.

- *Provide lots of praise*—The herculean work that's being done deserves high praise. Point out the pioneering nature of it, and the persistence required. Reinforce the courage that's come forth, and the competence. Summarize progress often, and offer encouragement and reassurance for the road ahead.

Goals Ground the Counseling Relationship

Goals are the threads that tie together the many challenges identified with the strategies to address them. Goals also connect the issues that were addressed with the assessment of counseling efforts. Thus, goals are useful for both clinical and program evaluation (or research) purposes.

This section will talk about how goals can structure the counseling sessions. Chapter 11 will look at the process of getting participant feedback. Chapter 13 will illustrate how goals were used to determine the helpfulness of counseling in this particular grant project. Please also refer to Chapter 13 for an explanation of the development and attribution of the goal-setting and evaluation tool.

Working with PWESD, then, the counselor uses the Framework for Coping with Early Dementia to explore concerns, develop goals, and monitor and review progress. The heart of the approach is to organize a "counseling care plan" according to the three domains of Emotional Adjustment, Practical Coping Strategies, and Lifestyle Issues. Each of the eighteen subheadings becomes a potential goal, as we saw when we went over all the challenges in Chapter 3. The list of goals presented in each domain is not all-inclusive, but rather, summarizes areas that may need attention. Figure 5.2 lays out a form for setting goals for your review and reference.

Early-Stage Alzheimer's Disease Counseling Goals

	Concerned	Already Addressing	Not Concerned
Emotional Adjustment:			
Understanding, acknowledging, and becoming more accepting of my condition			
Working toward finding new meaning/purpose in life			
Redefining my identity and feeling good about who I am			
Expressing feelings (both positive and negative) about my situation			
Having an attitude of being strong and capable			
Letting other people know that I want to be treated with respect			
Practical Coping Strategies:			
Learning and using stress management techniques			
Using memory aids and strategies			
Enhancing my ability to communicate, and informing others about it			
Paying more attention to physical exercise, diet, rest, and general health			
Doing memory and other cognitive exercise activities			
Getting emotional support from others			
Lifestyle Issues:			
Doing and/or developing new social and vocational activities			
Talking about and making future legal, financial, health, and care planning decisions			

(continued)

Figure 5.2.   Early-Stage Alzheimer's Disease Counseling Goals (Copyright © 2011, by Robyn Yale)

Acknowledging and working on challenges and changes with my family			
Asking for and accepting help from others			
Using early-stage support services			
Taking steps to problem-solve safety issues such as driving or managing finances			
Any Other Concerns?			
Top Goal Priorities			

Figure 5.2.   Early-Stage Alzheimer's Disease Counseling Goals (continued)

Determining and Setting Goals

Each person's goals will be unique. Goals may be selected in only one area, such as all emotional; or there may be a mix, such as emotional/practical or practical/lifestyle. It's not necessary or even feasible for every person to work in every area—individuals just choose what they want to focus on. Yet, goals are typically interrelated, so while a PWESD may be talking about only one of the three domains, a counselor who keeps the impact on the other two in mind is likely to be more effective.

Let's take an example. Person A sets a goal around replacing leisure activities he can no longer participate in, which is a lifestyle issue. While working to find new things he enjoys doing, you may also explore the emotional component, such as how he feels about the loss of previous identity and capabilities. You might also ask whether cognitive exercise is of interest as a new pursuit, which is one of the practical strategies. And, connecting him with an early-stage support group (from the lifestyle category) to reduce isolation again "cross-pollinates" the domains.

In another example, Person B selects understanding the disease as a primary goal. While receiving education and support from you as she works toward acceptance of her condition is an emotional task, she may disclose related family conflict along the way (categorized here with lifestyle). At the same time, she may be able to acknowledge how difficult it has become to manage some of the stresses caused by her symptoms (a practical coping strategy).

As you can see, goals are not linear. Rather, they are quite complex and multifaceted. Using the Framework helps to introduce, categorize, and prioritize a range of issues, thus making them more manageable. Goals can be thought of as touchstones to help people feel safe, comfortable, and in control enough to trust letting go into the counseling process. Goals are valuable for PWESD to envision and work toward a different future than they may have anticipated upon learning that their diagnosis was AD. In providing direction for counseling sessions as well as for efforts in one's life, goals are guideposts, which can also spark the energy and motivation needed to work on them.

When Are Goals Set?

Chapter 10 will describe in detail the protocol for initially assessing whether people are suitable for counseling. Goal setting takes place after phone screening, intake, in-person PWESD and family interviewing, and consent or agreement to begin counseling have all been obtained. So, the goals are discussed in your first session, by introducing the form provided in Figure 5.2. This separates them out from the task and distraction of paperwork occupying the previous encounters. It helps frame the counseling, setting the tone and stage. Goals can then be fresh in mind and at the ready, which also helps to cement the initiation of the therapeutic relationship.

How Are Goals Set?

From your initial assessment process, you have a sense of the person's concerns. This prior knowledge facilitates opening discussion about the choices on the goal sheet. For research purposes, it would be necessary to systematically go over and determine the level of interest in each option (and the rating system would need refinement). For clinical purposes, goals can flow more naturally from the conversation at hand.

It's important to make sure that the goal options are well understood. Reading and comprehension ability vary, so while the person should have the form in hand it's best to do more than have him or her fill it out. Going over the choices verbally and raising those that seem relevant but don't come up is a better way to proceed. The counselor then puts the concerns into the framework, filling out the checklist.

While having eighteen options seems like a lot for both PWESD and counselors, the three main domains (emotional, practical, lifestyle) are the organizing principle. You can suggest that PWESD pick their top one or two goals to work on. But, you don't want to limit them if multiple areas are of interest. On the other hand, structure is very helpful, and having too many goals can be unwieldy. Thus, the model is flexible, and you want to seek a balance between the extremes of confining the focus and having no focus at all. Ultimately, goals should be prioritized according to the issues of most importance. How many goals are finally set depends upon these priorities and the time you have to work together.

Goals may also change as counseling proceeds. Easier ones may be achieved and new ones may arise. Priorities can shift as part of the process. You might calibrate your counseling plan, then, as the person's interests and needs are clarified. For example, someone who wants to start by learning more about the disease may then be able to move into talking about feelings, or planning for the future.

Finally, some things may come up—initially or later—that aren't on the goal list. And, your skills may occasionally be called upon to artfully weave past life issues into discussion of the current situation if they arise. While you can't ignore these, you don't want to get "hijacked" by them either. You can gently guide the focus back to coping with early dementia as appropriate.

Thus, the goal-setting form is a work in progress, used as a tool as you go along. The counselor summarizes the major issues, gives the PWESD a copy to refer to, and explains that this will be the architecture of your work together. From here, you can construct a plan to work toward attaining the selected outcomes in your upcoming sessions.

Evaluating Progress toward Goals and the Counseling Sessions

Asking participants for feedback at the end of counseling provides valuable data about the impact of the intervention. Reviewing progress toward goals assesses whether people feel validated, and like they are coping better with early dementia. This is also an opportunity to ask about satisfaction with the counseling relationship and process.

A second form has been developed for use at this stage. However, rather than digress to the issues around evaluation and measurement of goal outcomes here, we will continue that discussion when we get to other administrative topics in Chapter 11.

Now that we've talked about this first step of setting goals, we'll next dive into addressing the special challenges faced by PWESD.

Addressing the Special Issues and Challenges Facing People with Early-Stage Dementia

All of the threads in our tale trace back to the point of sitting down and being present with the person with dementia to address the special issues he or she is facing. We're now at the apex then, of reentering the eighteen-point Framework for Coping with Early Dementia—this time with an eye toward intervention. Synthesizing the various elements we've been considering, we'll move forward by combining what we've learned so far: Understanding the various challenges that people may come in with, we build the counseling relationship, and begin the therapeutic process.

It isn't possible to include in what follows every possible way to work with every potential issue. You'll draw upon your own intuition, skills, and style. You'll assess each individual's situation and what the person brings to your alliance. And you'll have the formation of the framework to organize what occurs overtly with the other concerns of which you become aware.

Addressing Challenges

Part 1—A Framework for Coping: Emotional Adjustment

In this arena, the PWESD's task is to explore and integrate the psychological re-verberations (within oneself as well as with others) of being told that one has AD.

The emotional domain of coping helps individuals identify, express, and work through their feelings about the illness and all the different issues and challenges they are facing, as illustrated once again in Figure 6.1.

A. Acceptance of Condition

Let's look at the different aspects of accepting that one's condition is AD.

Understanding the Disease

In order to most effectively help, the counselor needs to find out where the person is in understanding and accepting the illness, because that will color any emotional responses. This is a process, rather than a fixed point. People may be either actively seeking or simply receptive to information, and if so, we can provide education and answer any questions they raise. For example, in early-stage support groups, participants typically want to discuss how the diagnosis of AD is determined; an explanation of the symptoms, course, and potential treatments; the latest research; and what to expect—both now and later.[1] The mystery of individual variability in the expression of the disease must be conveyed, while at the same time there are many developments known to be common to all PWESD. The distinction between AD, MCI, and other diagnoses will also need explicit clarification.

It can be tricky to talk with people directly about the disease as it can be quite sobering. Yet, there are ways to do it effectively—and it is our task to empower our clients. Chapter 10 will look at techniques of engagement from the point of first contact with a PWESD. After this initial screening process we can be assured that the person is coming to counseling to gain a better understanding. We offer it through the three domains of emotional support, coping with day-to-day practical issues, and looking at the impact on overall lifestyle. We strike the difficult balance between correcting any misconceptions (e.g., *does this mean that I won't know who my wife is next month?*) and providing honest appraisal of the possibilities (*this probably won't happen next month, but could at some point down the line*). When we

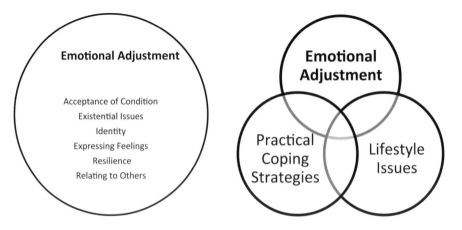

Figure 6.1. A Framework for Coping: Emotional Adjustment (Copyright © 2011, by Robyn Yale)

provide information we can do it sensitively and purposefully. For example: *It's true that there is now no cure for AD; but since the rate of each individual's progression is unknown, you may have much time ahead with high functioning and a good quality of life. How can we make that time as good as possible for you? What supports, activities, and relationships will help you to function at your best and feel most fulfilled? On the other hand, what do you need to think about and put into place in case decline occurs sooner rather than later? And how does everything you are learning and discussing here make you feel?*

Acknowledgment of Condition

Here it is helpful to explore what the experience of being diagnosed and dealing with medical professionals was like. Were individuals included in the discussion of evaluation results? Were they spoken with directly, kindly, and respectfully? Or, were they excluded, hurried, or avoided? Has their family talked with them about the illness or do they dance around it? Have they had the opportunity to process information and feelings? To what extent have they told friends, relatives, co-workers (if any), or others about their condition? Have they been wanting to do so but unsure whether or how to? What do they need before proceeding, and what will happen after they do? How do they usually handle complex challenges—alone, or by sharing with others?

Some people may still be reading about the illness, questioning or resisting their diagnosis even though they've agreed to be in counseling. Examining and talking with you about it at this time of uncertainty could be for some the main thing you and they accomplish together.

Acceptance

We want to allow the gradual and gentle process of "coming to terms" with having dementia. Where is this particular individual at in working through the situation, and does it change from session to session with you over time, rather than happen in a straight line? Establishing trust affords people opportunities to admit things they didn't before, and plenty of time to deal with their feelings and concerns. Let them know that you are unwaveringly here for them and that you appreciate how difficult this is. Praise their courage in facing their circumstances. Gird each step along the way with positive reinforcement. And help to offset the emotional trauma by letting them know you will also tackle the practical and lifestyle ramifications of acceptance.

A Special Note About Denial: Discussion of denial is woven into various chapters because it comes up in various contexts and at different points in the process. It is an issue for PWESD (Chapter 3); a "teaching" about counseling dynamics (Chapter 4); and can occur from the point of screening for counseling (Chapter 10) throughout intervention. Here let us say that it is never good to try to force those who are in denial out of that stance. At the same time, their first response or resistance is not always where they will stay. We must patiently allow vacillations, testing, and debating about the diagnosis *without pushing* for acceptance. This gives people slow and steady access to all of their contradictory feelings, and to your tenacious support. Here's an example: *It's ok that today you don't think you've had trouble with your checkbook. But you may not remember that you told me last time we met that this has happened a few times. Maybe we can revisit this and see if it becomes more troubling by the next time we talk about it, or not.* Then, in the next session you can say, *One time we met you said that managing your checkbook isn't a problem for you, but other times you've said that it can be. Sometimes this happens with memory loss—perceptions can change. How do you see this issue today—has anything about your checkbook come up in the past week?* While it is possible that disclosure and discussion about dementia will be traumatic, it can also be constructive. The unfortunate truth is that cognitive decline will occur whether it is acknowledged or not. The choice that PWESD along with their family and professional care partners have is whether to enable silence and denial or facilitate the emotional work that can engender resilience and healthy coping. Too often, the situation is as shown in Figure 6.2.

We end this critical section by restating it as a goal for the evaluation section that's ahead:

GOAL: Understanding, acknowledging, and becoming more accepting of my condition

B. Existential Issues

All of us occasionally contemplate such universal questions as the meaning of life or the journey of death. At times of crisis, the search for answers becomes even more compelling. Spiritual beliefs are often comforting and grounding. Counselors can engage PWESD in turning to those that are familiar, or cultivating new ones. Faith is sure to be tested as one confronts whether to struggle against reality or surrender to it. Having someone with whom to investigate and reflect upon these matters can be extremely helpful.

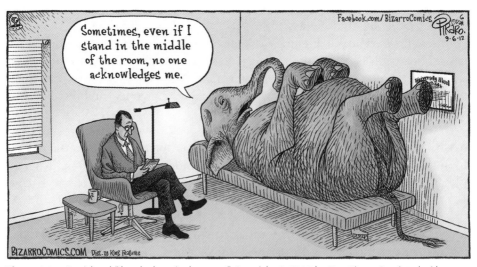

Figure 6.2. Denial and "the elephant in the room." Copyright © 2012 by Dan Piraro. Reprinted with permission.

Here we can discuss disease progression in light of spiritual traditions that bring solace. For example, one person with dementia wrote about practicing mindfulness, which attempts to keep the focus on the present moment more than on the past or future.[2] Others use religious institutions or literature, twelve-step programs, or support groups to find their way through this odyssey.

The counselor may help PWESD negotiate with others around issues of autonomy and independence. Even while making concrete arrangements, we facilitate the expression of their voices, wishes, and preferences. Reaffirming worth and personhood, we attempt to uphold dignity. And, from our vantage point here of emotional adjustment, note that it's important to deal with the feelings around these losses and the acceptance of new circumstances.

If there are simultaneous changes to address due to other age-related or health conditions, it's important to acknowledge these as well. Examples include sensory decline or limitations in mobility that affect what one can do.

And finally, people may be examining what their life purpose is while so much that was familiar evaporates. We'll talk more later about replacing lost roles and activities with new ones. Here we focus more on the internal process that accompanies this task. This brings us back to a central goal:

> **GOAL:** Working toward finding new meaning and purpose in life

C. Identity

Although abilities and independence are affected by dementia, people can rebuild from its assault on their sense of self. Counselors represent the view that the illness is disconnected from one's worth or value. For example, a person with diabetes wouldn't feel at fault or stupid. Similarly, the condition of dementia is not the sum total of who one is. Stereotypes can be explored and refuted, and more positive attitudes practiced. We can help people find things that they like about themselves or that others like about them, and things they are still good at doing. We can convey that the hard work of self-reflection and learning new coping skills to manage daily life with dementia is actually quite heroic.

We all go through the normal developmental process of consolidating our past, present, and future selves as the years go by. This is even more poignant with dementia since the natural flow of the task is interrupted. Facilitating grief work about what has passed, examining what remains, and looking optimistically at what might be born anew at this time serves to integrate a new sense of self. Reminiscence and life review allow people to discuss their previous successes, and how definitions of success might change as one ages and becomes more impaired. Articulating one's legacy can serve to reframe identity as not just being about what one does or achieves—but also about the kind of person one is. This blend of acknowledging what is no longer possible yet affirming hope for the future is a fundamental technique in the counselor's toolbox. It is certainly useful in working on this goal:

> **GOAL:** Redefining my identity and feeling good about who I am

D. Expressing Feelings

One of our biggest gifts as a counselor is offering our clients the opportunity to grieve. This process is usually roiled by erratic waves, rather than proceeding in a linear way. We allow the expression of a range of intense feelings and emotional reactions, knowing that all individuals go through it differently. They may or may not have experience with opening up to discuss such private matters with someone else. Respectful of this, we explore with care—with those who would like to—what it's like to lose one's competencies, one's dreams, one's vision of what life would hold.

Note that here it's also important to assess for clinical depression and suicidal ideation, and obtain outside mental health consultation if that would be appropriate. However, as PWESD talk and work through their issues and feelings they begin to metabolize the news of the diagnosis and all that it implies. They draw strength from the counselor's calm and unwavering presence.

Learning that one can survive this diagnosis, people begin to cultivate optimism and other positive feelings. Acknowledging the illness, they can expand the focus to the wellness that also exists, and often express relief and gratitude for this shift in perspective. The support of others and finding fulfilling activities and relationships are examples of unexpected areas of newfound appreciation. This brings us to our next goal:

> **GOAL:** Expressing feelings (both positive and negative) about my situation

E. Resilience

The definition of resilience in our current context is the positive capacity to withstand stress and regain one's buoyancy and good spirits. Helping people find and use their inner strength, confidence, and courage promotes renewal and a sense that life can go on. Despite the tragedy of the dementia diagnosis, one can reframe one's attitude to nurture empowerment and vitality. Coming to terms with the way things are over time permits a letting go and moving on—emotionally, in practical matters, and as regards one's overall lifestyle. Thus, here we reach a goal that sets an important foundation:

> **GOAL:** Having an attitude of being strong and capable

F. Relating to Others

Here the counselor lets PWESD know they can internally transmute negative views that people hold of them. In turn, PWESD can educate others in their lives about how they want to be perceived and treated. Even the act of teaching friends and family how they are experiencing dementia can serve to redefine a person's competence. Saying things like, *I'm still here, I'm able to do [this thing], I'm doing my best, I need more time to complete this, I want to be included in that discussion* is radical for those who would otherwise internalize all beliefs about being immediately incapacitated.

Of course, there will be times that PWESD need to give up control in some areas, and this is very difficult. But it doesn't have to mean that that happens completely, all at once, or in every area—and this needs to be understood. And, when it happens it can be done with consideration for the person's feelings. We'll talk a bit more about this later in this chapter. For now, we focus on this goal:

> **GOAL:** Letting other people know that I want to be treated with respect

Addressing Challenges

Part 2—A Framework for Coping: Practical Coping Strategies

The practical domain of coping helps people compensate for and adapt to their difficulties through the use of specific techniques and strategies. While cognitive impairment certainly alters the landscape of daily life, people can learn to manage the symptoms with attention to body and brain health. You will see as we go along that there is an interplay between these issues and the emotional adjustment discussed earlier in the chapter. Also, because many books and resources are available on each of these topics if you need them, what follows is simply a summary. The main point here is to be sure you are aware of the different elements included in this part of the framework, which you can see in Figure 6.3.

A. Stress Management

There are lots of strategies counselors can offer around managing the stress of having dementia. Many have been discussed in early-stage support groups, and literature written by PWESD affirms the helpfulness of those mentioned here.[3]

Perhaps the most important technique is adjusting one's attitude to the extent possible. This encompasses lowering expectations (of oneself and of others) about the pace or amount or types of things one can accomplish. It also means

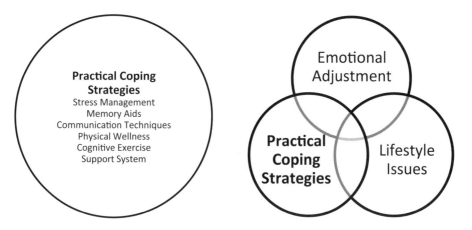

Figure 6.3.   A Framework for Coping: Practical Coping Strategies (Copyright © 2011, by Robyn Yale)

being kind, gentle, and patient with oneself rather than harsh and angry. Maintaining optimal mental health through talking to others (friends, family, and/or professionals), turning to spiritual faith, and trying to retain positive thinking even while acknowledging limitations are all relevant here.

Another primary suggestion in this area is to look at how things might be simplified. Slowing down, allowing more time for whatever is challenging, doing one thing at a time and with few distractions are all examples of this. Having structure with a predictable routine; a balance of enjoyable activities with tasks that are simply necessary; and built-in breaks can all help to keep the day calm.

There are also products and design considerations that can modify the safety of the home environment. For example, keeping walking paths clear and removing potentially hazardous materials and objects reduce accidents. New technology is being developed all the time now to assist people with tracking and tasks. Professionals specialized in this area can help families with dementia review various options.[4]

Other tools for managing stress include the healing power of humor, amazingly therapeutic bonds with pets, and the importance of relaxation. Deep breathing and meditation are skills that can be taught and practiced.

Lastly, it is important to mention that it's often tempting to cope with stress in unhealthy ways like alcohol or drug abuse, overeating, or other addictions. People with early dementia, like anyone else, can work toward modifying these habits and learn more nourishing ways to cope. All of this leads us to our next goal:

> **GOAL:** Learning and using stress management techniques

B. Memory Loss

The counselor helps the person find the best tools for his or her situation (while also addressing the feelings that the challenges are causing, such as frustration and stress—here we see the overlap of the dimensions of coping). PWESD benefit from education around practical strategies and assistive devices that can help them adjust to living with the constant forgetfulness. Memory aids to suggest include calendars for appointments and events, lists to help remember things to take care of, and use of an erasable whiteboard for other reminders. Setting up daily or weekly pill organizers and other medication-management systems are important for staying on schedule with what's been prescribed, as is a watch with an alarm. Some people prefer a home phone with big buttons and pictures of people often called, while others are able to manage cell phones and newer electronic equipment. A memory box or book with photos and other meaningful items can be comforting to PWESD who are becoming disoriented about the recent past. A preprinted business-size card saying something like "I have early dementia— thank you for your patience" can be given to restaurant or store personnel to reduce anxiety in those situations.

Counselors can also think through with the person how things can be better organized, for example offering tips for consistently putting certain things in certain places. Technology like a GPS reduces getting lost, if the person can use it. Mnemonics are also helpful for dealing with memory loss. Again, this is just a small sampling of available ideas. The Alzheimer's Association and similar organizations have many excellent resources and references to turn to in this area.

On another note, people can explore whether they might want to enroll in a clinical trial to see if experimental medication is effective for them. Also, more can be found in Chapter 4 about how you might navigate around memory loss (and communication—discussed next) in the counseling sessions. Here, PWESD have this goal:

GOAL: Using memory aids and strategies

C. Communication

Here we can explore with PWESD what makes communication easier or harder, and how they in turn can educate people in their lives about what they learn. For example, requesting that others speak more slowly and about one thing at a time is helpful. PWESD can also ask others to be patient and attentive in their listening, to refrain from interrupting, and to understand that more time may be needed to process thoughts and communicate them.[5] Letting people know whether or not they want assistance when words falter is a way to feel more in control rather than helpless at those times.

There are also techniques like "word substitution" that can be used when finding the right word is difficult. Again, the dementia care literature and organizations have much to offer about ways to enhance communication with PWESD, while also being respectful. And, we have to support the person around feeling upset when this happens in verbal interactions. Our goal here, then, is as follows:

GOAL: Enhancing my ability to communicate and informing others about it

D. Physical Wellness

Our role here includes educating PWESD about the ways in which monitoring and maintaining physical wellness optimize emotional health as well as cognitive performance. Ongoing attention to any medical conditions in addition to dementia is a critical part of this.

A lot of information is available about "heart-healthy" diets, which are now believed to be good for brain health as well.[6] Examples include eating low-fat foods, those rich in antioxidants, and many fruits and vegetables.[7] Exercise also plays a role, and even mild movement produces benefits like increased circulation. A plan can be structured to improve nutrition and the amount of physical activity throughout the day or week.

The counselor can explore which other habits and lifestyle factors are contributing to wellness and which may be undermining it. Wellness will also affect and be affected by many other areas of the framework. The best possible overall health gives one strength and stamina to cope with all the other challenges. And, of course in turn, effective coping in the ways discussed raises the likelihood of good health. Thus, we have this important goal:

> **GOAL:** Paying more attention to physical exercise, diet, rest, and general health

E. Cognitive Exercise

Mental activity is like exercise for the brain in the same way that physical exercise benefits the body. But in both cases, it is important to find the right level of challenge and exertion. The counselor can offer suggestions and resources while also supporting individuals who are discouraged by their limitations. Again, nothing can yet cure AD, but stimulation in the form of reading, puzzles, and games may enhance cognitive functioning for some people. Everyone with AD is different in terms of capabilities and interests, so individual assessment of the best "workout" is necessary. Training on the computer, classes, and cultural outings are examples of activities that may not appeal to or be easy for everyone. There is a good deal of expertise to refer to and tap for ideas about brain fitness.[8] This can help us steer the person toward this useful goal:

> **GOAL:** Doing memory and other cognitive exercise activities

F. Support System

The counselor's task here is to help PWESD build more of a social network to decrease feeling alone, and in particular to share with others what they are going through. We can explore whether support is likely to come from existing friends, family, involved professionals, or social contacts. And we can look into new sources such as other PWESD or early-stage support groups. Outlets for validation by and connection with others are good for mental, physical, and cognitive health as well. This can be summarized into a goal:

> **GOAL:** Getting emotional support from others

Addressing Challenges

Part 3—A Framework for Coping: Lifestyle Issues

In the lifestyle domain of coping, the counselor assists PWESD in recognizing and addressing changes that are currently happening as well as those that may

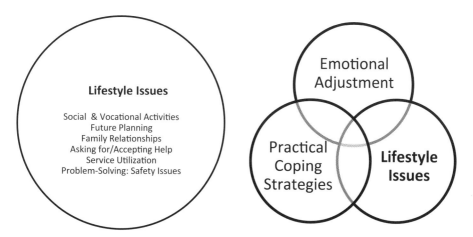

Figure 6.4   A Framework for Coping: Lifestyle Issues (Copyright © 2011, by Robyn Yale)

be necessary as the disease progresses, which are represented in Figure 6.4. As mentioned, the emotional and practical implications discussed earlier inextricably entwine with all of these complex issues. While many represent huge losses, there may also be gains in terms of new activities, improved relationships, helpful resources, and a sense of participation and control in the planning process.

A. Social and Vocational Activities

The counselor's task here is to help people examine the activities they are involved in, determine whether they can be maintained, and explore replacing those that can't with new ones. Part of this requires tough "letting go," while another part encourages holding on and rebuilding. This process is a central theme throughout our counseling work.

People with dementia have spoken and written about the possibility of having a life that includes fun, balance, growth, and contribution despite cognitive, physical, emotional, and social challenges.[9] Some recreational and/or work-related pursuits are likely to become less possible to do. Working through grief and toward acceptance is called upon here. But in other situations, finding new ways to accomplish tasks and activities successfully can empower people and boost their morale. For example, a person who formerly drove once a week to meet with friends but who can no longer drive may choose to get a ride rather than stop going. A person with a certain role in a social club may still be able to attend even if he or she doesn't perform the same function. If the hobby of reading becomes troublesome, audiobooks might be enjoyable. So creative adaptation is one skill we can offer to PWESD in hopes that they can sustain some of their leisure pursuits.

There are many new avenues to consider for spending time in structured and meaningful ways. Asking people about their interests, goals, and values; what makes them happy or stimulates them can unfold fresh perspectives and possibilities. Some have newly developed a hobby or discovered a talent or appreciation in the arts. Others have joined senior or adult day or early-stage programs that offer cultural outings, camaraderie, and community. Volunteer work is an option in many areas, and some do it by providing peer support to others with early dementia. And many have become part of the early-stage "movement," joining in advocacy and activism efforts. Whether small or large in scope, the individualized counseling approach allows people to design a new pattern to fit their own changing circumstances.

In the work world, modifying responsibilities is sometimes an option. If it isn't and a job has to end, the loss will ripple into one's identity, relationships, roles, and activities. Strategizing around telling an employer about the diagnosis of dementia and the resulting transition at work will be a key area of support. Advising or referring people for assistance with the change in financial status and applying for benefits to which they may be entitled is an area of expertise offered by the Alzheimer's Association and similar organizations.

This concise description of a very broad lifestyle issue can be summarized with the goal of:

GOAL: Doing and/or developing new social and vocational activities

B. Future Planning

While a person is still in the early stage, it is important to expediently deal with legal, financial, and health care planning issues. At this perilous time of so much in flux, the counselor can provide education and clarity about what matters need attention and why they must be addressed now. If PWESD have not executed wills, trusts, powers of attorney, and advance health care directives, they need to do so while still competent to make and implement those decisions.

Estate planning, to protect and administer one's assets upon incapacity or death, requires consultation with a specialized elder law attorney. A financial planner and/or care manager can help to sort out the impact of a job ending on existing resources, and advise about applying for Social Security disability, Veterans Administration, or other benefits. Loss of income and insurance must also be analyzed in light of the huge potential costs if long-term care is required in the future. Exploring and anticipating services that may be needed and a possible change in living situation are also part of the picture here.

Discussing who to designate to make medical and financial decisions in the event that one is no longer able to—and how these affairs will be managed as dementia progresses before incapacity—are enormous conversations. Resources, relationships, and preferences must all be examined. Counseling may or may not be the place to tackle all of it, but raising the issues is vital. Again, organizations like the Alzheimer's Association, Alzheimer's Foundation of America, Alzheimer's Disease Education and Referral Center, and AARP have excellent literature, expertise, and links to local professionals who can assist in these various areas.

Coming to terms with the likelihood of future incapacity while still in the process of accepting current early-stage impairments is a challenging conundrum. Striving to believe that a full, positive life can continue with mild dementia while facing inevitable future decline further complicates the paradox. Through it all, the counselor must be sensitive to the emotional tasks involved as well as the tactical ones—for example, asking what it feels like to be contemplating and metabolizing these weighty matters.

Lastly, one lawyer with dementia wrote an article suggesting that, while PWESD need to put future plans in place, they shouldn't obsess so much that they don't live the life they still have in the present—wise counsel indeed![10] This goal, then, encompasses a number of balancing acts:

> **GOAL:** Talking about and making future legal, financial, health, and care-planning decisions

C. Family Relationships

In the vast arena of family relationships, we explore shifting roles and responsibilities that need attention. The many inevitable changes are typically accompanied by a sense of grief and loss as well as confusion about adjustments that need to be made. The counselor helps PWESD articulate their issues and feelings, prepare to talk with their families, and advocate for themselves when it is possible.

You may recall that, in other pieces of the framework, we talked about fortifying PWESD to educate others about stigma and about communication strategies. In this context, we see that the therapeutic benefits of family involvement can include diagnosed individuals feeling empowered to represent their own views.[11] Ideally—and this is why early intervention is so critical—we tackle issues before there is a full-blown crisis. PWESD need encouragement to feel confident, as well as opportunities to participate in decision making and planning. Rapport with the counselor can be more important than the content of the session when helping PWESD express values and care preferences to their family members.[12]

Families will have previous patterns of relating and other circumstances coexisting with the dementia, making each family you encounter unique and complex. In addition to the challenges they face, many are able to find gifts for which to be grateful, such as slowing down and prioritizing, or appreciating mutual strengths and support.

Chapter 7 will talk more about how family issues fit into the three domains of the coping framework. For now we will summarize with this goal:

> **GOAL:** Acknowledging and working on challenges and changes with my family

D. Asking for/Accepting Help

There are many ways in which PWESD may now need assistance with initiating and executing tasks. Consenting to receive help from others, though, does not come easily for everyone. Offering it respectfully and with an effort to preserve the person's dignity are important here. The counselor facilitates the understanding that what PWESD are experiencing is due to the illness, in hopes of reducing embarrassment, guilt, and fear.[13] And, helping people to admit that they are making mistakes or recognize that things are becoming harder to do may ease the discomfort of high expectations. Reframing assistance as a way to preserve optimum functioning and put new supports in place puts it in the context of improvement rather than debilitation. Help can also be offered and accepted in steps, instead of in multiple areas and all at once.[14] Once again, we come upon the balance of holding on and letting go. As the person works on the many other pieces of the framework, we arrive at the next goal:

GOAL: Asking for and accepting help from others

E. Service Utilization

Here, the counselor assists PWESD to explore and enroll in early-stage AD and other relevant programs. Part of this is working through concerns about using services. Another piece is to learn about what is available now as well as over time. Then, the person (and family) can begin accessing resources that will serve them well throughout the inevitable transitions between levels of care that are likely to occur in the future.

Some regions have developed more early-stage programs than others. Many now have early-stage support groups for the diagnosed person, which provide camaraderie while helping them understand and cope with the illness.[15] Senior and adult day centers may have appropriate components to their programs. In some areas, a wealth of innovative activities exist, offering cultural outings, artistic expression, theater, singing, and other pleasurable pursuits.

For those who don't prefer group experiences, hiring a companion is an option. Others take advantage of telephone support from early-stage peers. In educational events put on by Alzheimer's organizations, people can learn about the disease, local resources, and clinical trials of experimental medications. Dementia care agencies now have technological advancements, such as social networking, private chats, and message boards. And before too long, it is hoped that it will be easy to find ongoing individual counseling for PWESD and their families! From now forward, this goal provides a service within a service:

GOAL: Using early-stage support services

F. Problem-Solving: Safety Issues

Safety issues are serious, and they need to be confronted. With each person and situation, however, there may be solutions that support independent functioning for a period of time. And, when that isn't possible, alternatives can be sought to substitute for what is being taken away.

For example, the counselor educates the person about how dementia impacts driving. Combining this factual information with talking through feelings of grief and loss may lower resistance to the idea that driving can be problematic. When PWESD are able to come to the decision to stop driving themselves, it spares the family the pain of imposing this. Professional driving assessments help to determine when this is necessary. Sometimes recommendations are made to reduce the distance traveled, but not completely cease driving for a while. When driving does need to stop, strategizing about transportation is helpful, such as getting rides from others or using a ride service. The Alzheimer's organizations often mentioned here have useful information about this whole area, and there is also abundant relevant literature.[16]

As far as managing finances, once again there may be steps taken to preserve autonomy, such as having family or professional help with only certain rather than all aspects. For instance, checks can be prepared for the person to sign. The counselor can help the person and family identify which parts of this huge task are problematic, organize systems, and suggest resources to get a handle on them.

Safety issues around being home and going out alone also need to be assessed and analyzed. In-home, companion, meals, or early-stage program services may alleviate some concerns. There are ways to continue enjoying cooking when it becomes difficult, such as being part of preparing a meal without having the sole responsibility, or watching food-related television shows. Pillboxes and watch alarms can remind people about medication, and there are many other safety-related products on the market. Identification bracelets are important before getting lost becomes a concern.

Of course, more supervision is needed in these and many other areas as time goes along. The point here is to involve PWESD in changes when possible through acknowledgment, explanation, exploration of feelings, and decision making. The counselor will likely be negotiating varying points of view within the family, while being an advocate for the person with dementia as appropriate.

By now it should be clear that problem-solving around safety also connects with such other areas of the framework as denial, existential issues, accepting help, and relating to others. Given this web of underpinnings, our last goal is very fitting:

> **GOAL:** Taking steps to problem-solve safety issues such as driving or managing finances

Addressing Challenges: Summary

We've now made our way through the pastiche of issues that make up the Framework for Coping with Early Dementia. As explained previously, the purpose was to raise awareness rather than to focus on the details of solving each area. We've also explored the trinity between building the counseling relationship, identifying challenges, and addressing them. We understand the need to proactively integrate the triad of tightly interwoven domains (emotional, practical, and lifestyle).

There is an art to focusing on present living without becoming overwhelmed by losses of the past or future. This represents yet a third trine: honoring who the person has always been, drawing forth the essence of who they are now, and anticipating who they might potentially become. It connects the counselor with the counselee, as they navigate through all the grave concerns as well as the optimistic hopes about what is yet to come.

The foundation and atmosphere of kindness set by the counselor show the PWESD a path to poignant self-acceptance. It's amazing but true that this fundamental human exchange can be the root of renewal and transformation, cutting through this twisted, terror-inducing disease. Leaving behind blame and judgment frees the person for the gifts of reflection, deepening inner wisdom, and self-actualization. Making connections between all the moving parts sparks an alchemy that constructively changes attitudes and behavior. In keeping with our initial theme of revolution and evolution, we can see how the ingenuity and valor of the counselor cultivate the strengths in each PWESD to battle and grow forward, however that needs to happen.

The Role of the Family

Transformation through Evolution and Revolution

While the person with early dementia is the central character in this tale, family members are certainly in a supporting role. Families were integral to the discussion around identifying and addressing challenges, and you have probably been wondering about them. Since there is a good deal of literature readily available about caregiving and dementia in general, we'll discuss that here only briefly. Then we'll go on to explore the dynamics between PWESD and their care partners. Finally, we'll focus more specifically on how family members can best be incorporated into this counseling service.

Families need to be—and in fact, are—part of everything we are doing here. Our practices with families are evolving, to incorporate PWESD in discussions and decisions where possible. Family relationships transform through adaptation and change as dementia takes hold; but as we will see, not always in only one direction. Despite potential and actual internal strife, families can be our allies in helping people face having the disease and overcoming stereotypes about it. Thus, families are also fierce warriors whose courage invaluably aids PWESD in achieving the victories of acceptance and new ways of coping.

Family Care Partners

Most people with early dementia live at home, and many have family members involved. Overall, more than 15 million Americans provide unpaid care to persons with Alzheimer's and other dementias, at an estimated economic value of $210.5 billion in 2011.[1] While PWESD usually don't yet require intensive direct care or supervision, their relatives are affected by, and usually play an extremely important role in, their new circumstances. There are a myriad of issues that may arise within a family after the diagnosis is determined, and they are distinct from what's at the forefront in the later stages of the disease.

In the pilot project described in Chapter 13, families participated to only a limited extent due to time and funding constraints. Likewise, your setting and resources will determine how much you can offer. Ideally, early-stage family care partners would also receive counseling, either separately and/or in joint sessions with their diagnosed relatives. There are many more general counseling services available to care partners than to PWESD, but there is still an urgent need for specialized training, expansion of services, and corresponding outcome research particular to the early stage. Readers with the requisite skills and interest are encouraged to hop aboard and take these on!

Care Partners and the Framework for Coping with Early Dementia

The three domains of coping that we discussed for PWESD apply to their family members as well. Care partners have to cope with their own feelings around the disease, the many daily practical issues that arise, and the need for future plans. Family systems are complex, and what happens to one member exponentially compounds shifts in relationships amongst all the others—whether they be spouses, siblings, parents, children, or other extended relatives.

The following list summarizes some of the many potential family issues:

Emotional Adjustment—As with individual PWESD, individual family members have their own unique response to the diagnosis of AD. They vary (and vacillate) in their level of understanding and acceptance of the disease. They may cope with denial initially or on an ongoing basis. There are many overwhelming feelings to process, such as grief, distress, anger, fear, and worry. They may or may not want to talk about the situation, often fearful of upsetting the PWESD and ashamed to tell others because of the stigma.

Practical Coping Strategies—Care partners often have their own physical, mental health, and other stresses in their lives in addition to those of the PWESD. There may also be dissension amongst family members if some don't want to accept or assist with the situation. Enabling the PWESD to function as well as possible is one challenge, and helping with the things that have become difficult for the PWESD to do is another. Additionally, families need to learn how to relate to their relative with dementia, including strategies to deal with memory and communication impairments.

Lifestyle Issues—There may be struggles with the PWESD around how and how much care partners should intervene with assistance and supervision due to differences in perception about what is going on. Negotiating concerns around safety (such as cooking or doing certain things alone) have to be balanced with respect for autonomy where it is possible. There may be changes in roles and dynamics within the family that are complicated by preexisting unresolved interpersonal issues. Many decisions must be made around legal and financial planning issues, and the coordination of care.

Care Partners Need to Address Their Own Issues

It is well known and heavily documented that caregiving can adversely affect the health of family members.[2] As one author put it, "All who give care need to take care."[3] Self-care helps relieve the many stresses of caregiving, which may be physical (e.g., exhaustion); emotional (e.g., depression); mental (e.g., boredom); social (e.g., isolation); occupational (e.g., absenteeism); and spiritual (e.g., loss of belief). Daily attention to body, mind, heart, and spirit can occur in the form of relaxing and nourishing practices along with the avoidance of unhealthy coping behaviors (like overusing alcohol).

Families also benefit, of course, from education and support around dementia. Fortunately, there are many excellent resources for care partners such as workshops, literature, support groups, online chats, and other services. Local and national dementia care organizations are excellent sources of information and referral.

Dynamics between PWESD and Their Care Partners

In previous chapters, we looked at the challenges facing PWESD through the lens of the coping framework, and strategies to address them. We saw that acknowledging and working on family issues was a central theme across all three domains. We talked, for example, about PWESD wanting to be treated with respect instead of being assumed to be incapacitated. And that relating to care partners involves exploring feelings and changes; reframing and redefining role expectations; and doing a good deal of negotiating to try to meet everyone's needs.

The early stage is a unique time for families. The focus can be on the present, rather than only on the long-term future; on strengths and not just deficits; and on involving rather than excluding the diagnosed person. PWESD who talk about their feelings and experiences can help to make problem-solving and planning decisions that affect them, and can still participate in other aspects of family life.

The counselor facilitates partnership, which empowers PWESD to engage in this process, and to be heard. The person and family each try to understand what it's like for the other, often becoming more tolerant, appreciating one another, and coping together as a team.[4]

Certainly, this is the best-case scenario! There might instead be a lot of conflict. Still, families can learn to intervene in ways that preserve the PWESD's sense of control and self-esteem. Allowing time rather than taking over, asking what help is needed, and letting some less important things go are all possibilities. New ways to do things can be found when care partners let their diagnosed relatives teach and guide them on how to best provide support.

PWESD can also learn to give care as well as receive it. Acknowledging and respecting the feelings of care partners, and finding ways to relieve care partners' stresses when possible are examples of this type of reciprocity.[5]

Many PWESD and families have been eminently able to transcend the heartache of the dementia experience together. For some, it's been a private process, while others have taken it into the public arena by writing, speaking, and advocating within the field. One son wrote about how the disinhibition caused by dementia brought down a lifelong wall of silence; his father expressed words of love he had always yearned to hear.[6] A gentleman with dementia wrote about what it's like for him now that his wife runs the home and family. While acutely aware and somewhat ashamed of the loss of his own role, he "still has other sides" to his life. He's contributed by authoring publications encouraging people with dementia to see that it doesn't have to be "all doom and gloom."[7]

Tyler Summit, the college-age son of legendary women's basketball coach Pat Summit, talked about his mother being diagnosed with early-onset AD in 2011. She revealed it publicly, and then kept working for some time with assistance and modifications to her previous role. Tyler says, "*My mom has definitely always been my role model. . . . Alzheimer's disease has just given me more ways to strive to be like [her]. Despite [it], she has stuck to her principles and stayed strong in her faith. Her confidence to be open about this disease has taught me the importance of honesty.*"[8]

As the early-stage field has evolved in some regions, programs for PWESD and families together have been developed. To name just a few, there are support groups for early-stage individuals with their spouses, cultural outings for groups of PWESD and families, and even a monthly social dance for couples!

As a last example, Alzheimer Europe just initiated a working group of eleven PWESD and care partners to advise the organization and ensure that their activities reflect the priorities and views of people with dementia.[9] More and more local, national, and international agencies are incorporating this type of coalition and input into their board structures, mission statements, and organizational agendas.

Care Partners and This Counseling Program

Although family counseling was not part of the pilot project described in Chapter 13, families were involved in a number of ways. They were included in the initial assessment process, occasionally invited into the end of the PWESD counseling sessions, and at least on some level stayed in communication with the counselors. Families need to be involved in discussions when termination is considered. They can also be part of your program evaluation or research protocol. And, of course, they are the critical link for carrying out the follow-up plan.

While family participation is ideal, for some it is not possible because they are too busy, stressed, or otherwise not available. Certain logistical matters may require a care partner's help, though, such as transportation to sessions, being an emergency contact, scheduling sessions, following up on suggested coping strategies, and linking to community resources. Whether care partners are present or not when PWESD are in counseling, it's important to know where they will be and how to reach them.

The counselor's relationship with the family begins at the point of screening and intake. Chapter 10 describes the protocol for gathering the PWESD's history. The family's needs are also explored during this interview process. Their input on the PWESD's issues opens the door to ongoing contact. However, care partners must understand that the PWESD is the focus of the service. The counselor has to be clear on the purpose of the program and set limits on family participation. For example, there may be preexisting marital issues that go beyond how dementia impacts the relationship. While difficult to tease apart, the focus here would be on the individual with dementia in the context of the couple's dynamics. You might also be drawing boundaries so that unrelated external issues don't dominate conversation.

At the same time, you want to maintain contact with care partners through periodic check-in by phone or meetings—depending on the latitude of your job. Perhaps it goes without saying, but as a reminder it's important not to talk in front of the PWESD as if he or she weren't there.

The way this is presented to the person and the family is important. A written agreement explaining the intent of the new program and discussing confidentiality is useful for clarifying parameters. A sample of this will be presented in Chapter 10.

The principle of confidentiality applies to PWESD as much as to any other person. Exceptions to this would be in matters of safety, emergencies, and mood or behavior changes warranting examination, or if there are issues that the PWESD gives the counselor permission to share with his or her family. Explaining that everything you discuss in counseling will be considered confidential with these exceptions, and being explicit about what the exceptions might be, is an important step in the enrollment process. General sharing about how the person is doing in counseling is acceptable, but for anything more specific, always ask permission before sharing information with family.

This counseling model has the advantage of being flexible, which is good because each family is so different from any other. There may be times when the PWESD chooses to have a care partner come in for the last ten to fifteen minutes of a counseling session. This is especially helpful when the counselor is sending the person home with memory aids or other tools to practice during the week.

It can also be used for expressing feelings, or updating family on lifestyle issues discussed. You may want to prepare in advance with the PWESD if you agree that it will be best to include the family. Given the short time frame, you'll need to be very brief and focused with them.

The best situation is if your setting enables you to have longer, joint counseling sessions with PWESD and their care partners, or to have supplemental counseling sessions for care partners so that their needs can be more fully addressed. Alternatively, hopefully there are other trained professionals to refer to in your region who can do this. Another option is for you to have family meetings with PWESD and as many relatives as are appropriate. Especially in this venue, it is likely that you'll have to orient everyone toward the topics the PWESD requests and around the dementia, in contrast to all the potential family issues. This has to be done in a kind and sensitive way, but for practical purposes there is only so much that can be tackled at any one time.

Lastly, you are the advocate for PWESD, since they are not likely to have any other. This doesn't have to mean that you are adversarial with family—it's just that your role is to insure that the PWESD's concerns are conveyed. In doing so, you also model for family care partners how to use constructive communication techniques and have calm and respectful interaction.

CHAPTER 8

Illustrating with Case Examples

Our tale can be illustrated by viewing case examples through the prism of the coping framework. Examining the multi-hued nuances of family constellations and dynamics in this way brings to life the clinical concepts and practices described thus far. The range of diverse scenarios, personality types and combinations of topics you could encounter is infinite, but a few are presented here for your consideration.

If you are a sole practitioner and/or have opportunities for peer consultation, case examples can be used to reflect upon how you might feel and respond across different intense and complex situations. If you are in a position to train others to be counselors, real or composite examples like these can be used in teaching workshops. Case examples can also be turned into role plays by describing the scenes and characters and rehearsing potential interactions. Those conducting training should have a solid clinical background and experience with this intervention.

Case examples can also be used to raise awareness and educate people who aren't in a direct role but would benefit from understanding the nature of the service. This might include other agency staff, collaborating professionals, and board members. And, the cases below take place in a few types of settings, in case you happen to be the referral person but not the actual counselor. There are a variety of entry points by which PWESD may find their way into counseling.

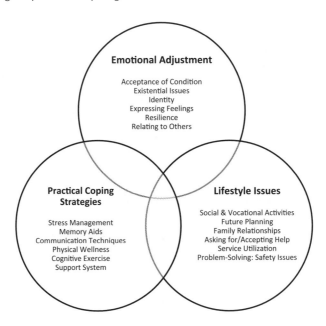

Figure 8.1. The Framework for Coping with Early Dementia (Copyright © 2011, by Robyn Yale)

As you review these cases, give some thought to how early intervention is different than what you might do in the mid-to-late stages of the disease. At the same time, watch for the edges of overlap with care management or other services that you'll often cross. Note, too, that some skills you use are typical of any counseling situation, and some are unique to this population. Trust your existing knowledge and skills while also staying open to new learning through this unique experience.

Some of the key things to look for include opportunities to balance discussion of loss and resilience; reframe the trauma of change with the positives in peoples' lives; find strengths and abilities that can be explored and developed; and pursue alternative strategies for achieving personal goals. For a quick refresher and for your reference as you proceed, Figure 8.1 contains the Framework for Coping with Early Dementia in its entirety.

Case #1—A True Story

Let's begin with the true story of Terry, whose partner Andrea (names have been changed) called me with concerns about Terry's driving. They had lived together for ten years but weren't married (which placed some constraints on actions she could take). I had the privilege of working with him for over a year, which is certainly not always the case. Sessions were with Terry alone, although Andrea was often asked to join us before we ended our meetings.

Terry had been told that his diagnosis was early-stage AD the month before but never mentioned it to anyone—including Andrea. The doctor had told Terry he'd be reporting the diagnosis to the Department of Motor Vehicles (DMV), and Andrea wanted him to "face reality." It often takes several months before the DMV responds with a notice to either come in for a driving test or cease driving. There is a lot of variability in how different DMVs across the country handle reports of diagnosis.

When I first met him, Terry was very pleasant and agreeable, but he wasn't convinced that he had AD and he sure didn't think it had anything to do with driving. I began by answering his questions about AD, including how the diagnosis was determined and whether anything he was experiencing might relate to it. I also explained the way dementia impacts driving, and he was quite sure he wasn't having any of those problems. I raised the idea that sometimes people didn't believe they had dementia because they didn't feel like the stereotype of a person who was completely incapacitated. He agreed with this, and, although it didn't immediately lessen his defensiveness, it seemed to register. I acknowledged his interest in learning about the disease and his willingness to talk with me.

Like most people, Terry was quite reliant on his car, felt he'd always been a good driver, and didn't want to give up his license. He also didn't want to burden Andrea with taking him everywhere he wanted to go. Over time he came to realize that she would actually be relieved of worry if she took over the driving, and that there were other ways to get around—including "my two good legs." We also explored using other options, like a transportation service and friends picking him up.

Eventually, Terry began to admit to me that he was concerned about memory "gaps," like having lost his car five or six times; and the "few times" he'd realized he wasn't paying attention while driving and had to pull over. He also acknowledged how stressful this was. He went through a period where he said he still planned to drive but understood his family's concern about it. But he said that if his license were taken away, he wouldn't drive.

Once when Andrea joined us in the session we wrote an agreement that limited his driving quite a bit to certain times and places. She expressed her willingness to do the driving, and he expressed his appreciation.

He did start driving less, but sometimes said he wanted to take the car out to "see how it feels." He promised to be more careful, and I explained that this wasn't something he could be sure of being able to control. We reviewed the safety risks and liabilities, the doctor's recommendation that he stop driving, and the effect of brain changes on his ability to observe himself while driving. Andrea was angry that he insisted on continuing to drive and wasn't facing his impairments, and the three of us talked about how acceptance can be slow because denial can fluctuate. When the DMV notice came requesting that he appear for a driving test he postponed going, admitting to "cold feet" and worry that he wouldn't pass. I reinforced the couple's positive efforts to work together through this difficult issue.

Meanwhile Terry had begun using other transportation options and could see that his life could continue without driving. When the notice later came to suspend his license, he wasn't happy about it but did gradually come to terms with it saying, *"I think you're really helping me. . . . I'm more amenable to things in my thoughts and actions. I'm through with driving, it's no longer part of who I am—it makes sense to me now. I no longer have to fight about it, even within myself. I feel cleansed."* Andrea was able to praise him for working things through in this way.

However—and this I found very interesting—acceptance around driving didn't translate to other areas. Andrea had been quite worried about Terry responding to too many sweepstakes offers and phony mail solicitations as well as losing two wallets and overlooking bills to be paid. Once again he at first denied any impairment, but before long could admit to me (not to her yet) that he'd always been careless with bookkeeping and was finding it even harder to keep it straight now. When Andrea joined us and suggested that she handle his mail, he said he felt demeaned because he had been in the advertising field and knew all about junk mail. But he was willing to take information from me about how to get off of solicitors' mailing lists.

Andrea was frustrated that it took an hour for Terry to write a check. Once again his first stated concern was that he didn't want to burden her with more things to do. We reviewed the doctor's recommendation that he should no longer handle banking, and the fact that memory loss makes it easy to overlook details and hard to complete tasks. Again we signed agreements, taking things in steps: one week saying she would open the mail and keep the bills in one place; later followed by deciding together when to pay them and her filing them when they were paid. They also limited the cash that was available for him to carry and tried using a money belt.

This went on for some time, progressing from their paying bills together to his gradually accepting her doing it. He wasn't happy about it—he didn't want to give up control. For awhile he insisted on continuing to write checks for charitable donations. But he understood her frustration and knew that his judgment could be affected. Finally he was able to admit this awareness to her and express gratitude for her help, saying, *"It's not easy to deal with someone who's not 100% with their memory."* The agreements only worked partially, but when we reviewed them he could see the need for them. I reminded them both that it was not his fault, and she was able to say that she understood how hard this was for him. I commended their teamwork, their open communication, their honesty; their forgiveness and kindness to one another; and their progress over time in terms of his letting go and her taking on more. I also supported his coming to terms with the loss of this role and ability especially so soon after the recent loss of driving.

In the meantime, since the start of our counseling sessions, we'd been looking at how Terry spent his time. He still played tennis but was finding it harder to enjoy adult education classes he'd always attended. I found a senior companion service that paired him with a person who knew photography and could take him out to pursue this hobby of his in an unpressured way. He also agreed to sign up for a cardiac exercise class that his doctor had recommended when he heard that it might also be good for his cognitive functioning. He and Andrea started going to concurrent early-stage support groups for PWESD and their care partners. Other areas we explored but he decided against included volunteer work, going to the local senior center, and doing some writing.

One day Terry said, *"I feel I have no central purpose. I have energy and intellect, I should offer something to society."* I had an upcoming speaking engagement at a national public affairs forum on political and social issues. I had been having PWESD speak at conference sessions and other venues with me for many years to provide a firsthand account of coping with AD and asked whether Terry and Andrea were interested in participating in this one. They agreed to do it and did it very well. An example of his remarks was, *"Alzheimer's doesn't throw me. I feel it cemented my relationship with Andrea. I still enjoy tennis, and though it was hard to give up driving I'm managing without it. I know that I'm in the early stage and it may get worse. I'm curious about the future but I don't dwell on it. I feel I'm doing well, and I'm in good spirits."* As you might imagine, the presentation was quite powerful and received very positive feedback. They also participated in a town hall meeting for PWESD and families hosted by the Alzheimer's Association.

Then, Andrea wanted to attend a caregiver respite event that would have her away from home for three days and two nights. She worked with the family consultant at the caregiver support agency to give herself permission to do this and arrange in-home care. I had been encouraging her to consider her own counseling as well for her worry and stress, but she hadn't followed up on that. I had additionally suggested a financial case manager, but she didn't want an outside person involved. The three of us had also talked about the fact that Terry had never designated powers of attorney, and he'd begun to see how urgent it had become. It took awhile but he eventually agreed for them to see an attorney and take care of that.

As the months went on, Terry began to have more memory lapses, which for some time he recognized and admitted. He wanted to know "how deep" I thought his disease was—when things would get worse, and what would happen over time. He at first resisted but ultimately agreed to wear an identification bracelet after getting turned around while walking in his neighborhood. I explained that the rate of decline was unpredictable and praised his courage in facing it and the steps he was taking. At one point he had his 85th birthday and we did some life review. A close friend had recently died and he was grateful for another birthday and reflected on having had a good life.

Eventually Terry began to feel he shouldn't stay at home so much, and Andrea was getting more stressed and anxious about her own health. He started going to an adult day program three times a week, where he benefited from the socialization and stimulation. He enjoyed attending, though he felt healthier than most others who were there. He was becoming less aware of his memory issues, and around this time we agreed to end our counseling relationship. Both of them expressed appreciation for the work we'd done, and I told them it had been meaningful to me as well.

I hope this description helps to illuminate the coping framework with its refraction of emotional, practical, and lifestyle issues. I couldn't make it a good thing that Terry had AD or make it go away. As with anything in life, they had to bear this misfortune and adjust to it, finding the resilience to go on. I tried to offer moments of quiet reflection amidst the upheaval for expressing feelings and answering questions. Acceptance of the disease didn't come in a straight line, and this narrative can't adequately describe the peaks and valleys of that emotional process. But Terry went from not wanting to tell anyone about his diagnosis to public speaking about it, as have many other PWESD. Even when his resistance or denial reappeared, he continued asking for information and assimilating his experiences. I tried to respect his pace and boundaries, and he seemed to feel trusting and comfortable. By the time the driver's license was revoked he was in a different place than he likely would have been if a counselor were first called at that time—because he'd received explanations and explored alternatives. Having a long-term relationship allowed us the luxury of time to touch upon most other areas of the framework, including communication, physical wellness, new activities, accepting help, using services, and family relationships. The couple's dynamics were in no way simple or straightforward, but they did manage to problem-solve a good deal together, learn strategies to cope with the disease, and see that they could handle its demanding transitions. The following year after terminating, when I learned that Terry had moved to residential care, I hoped that the quality of his life up to that point had been better than it might have been if we had never met.

Feel free to peruse the case and see if there are other things you might have done with Terry's situation. Think about how you might have felt dealing with the challenges of the counseling role. Next we are going to look at a few hypothetical, but potentially very real, additional cases.

Case #2—Assisted Living Resident

Let's say that you work or are called in to an assisted living community where a woman who moved in recently is isolating a lot and seems confused. Other residents often gossip and snicker about her. If you were to intervene, what would you do? Here are just two things from each domain of the eighteen-point framework (Figure 8.1) that I would think about. What else occurs to you?

Emotional

Acceptance of condition—Explore whether she's concerned about her confusion and has seen a doctor about it.

Expressing feelings—Ask how she's feeling about her recent move to this place—in terms of both losses and gains.

Practical

Communication techniques—See if the isolation might have to do with embarrassment around talking with others.

Memory aids—Discuss whether memory aids can help with confusion (e.g., keeping room key in a certain place).

Lifestyle

Social activities—Determine interests and activities available in the residence.

Problem-solving safety issues—Inquire about reassessing whether she has been provided with the appropriate level of care.

You could probably find most or even all areas of the framework relevant here, but you would have to prioritize with this person about her own goals. Depending on your own time and energy you could also go beyond the counseling role to offer such things as giving an educational talk to residents about memory loss; or consulting with staff about early dementia.

Case # 3—Mother and Daughter

In this situation, you work or are called by a social service agency with a caregiver support program. An adult daughter is quite angry and resentful, and her mother with dementia who now lives with her seems depressed. Again there are only two elements listed from each domain of the framework in the following list that might emerge or be considered. What else can you offer in beginning a counseling relationship with the mother?

Emotional

Identity—Explore how the mother's lifelong role with her daughter is affected by her having dementia.

Relating to others—See if she'd like to ask her daughter to talk to her in a kinder tone.

Practical

Stress management—Ask about the stress level in the home environment (and about risks of suicide or elder abuse).

Support system—Assess whether the mother has anyone to talk to for support.

Lifestyle

Future planning—Determine whether the family has done estate, legal, or long-term care planning.

Family relationships—Offer to meet with the mother and daughter together.

Once again, you can probably think of additional areas of the framework that might come into play. And, depending upon the limits of what you can provide beyond counseling, you could potentially extend support to the mother or to agency staff who are working with her.

Case #4—Spouse in Denial

Now you are working in or called by a memory disorders clinic. A man with early dementia seems relieved and accepting when told his diagnosis after the team evaluation, but his wife continues to insist that there is nothing wrong. She agrees to his counseling thinking it will make him "try harder." In addition to the remaining two points from each domain of the framework mentioned in the following list, how else might you handle this situation?

Emotional

Existential issues—Explore how the man is reevaluating himself and his life having received news of his diagnosis of AD.

Resilience—Build on his acceptance thus far by looking at what he'd like to put into place so that he feels his days are fulfilling.

Practical

Cognitive exercise—Ask whether he does or is interested in activities that stimulate the brain and memory (e.g., appropriate puzzles).

Physical wellness—Discuss the results of the rest of his medical evaluation and how he might best remain in good health.

Lifestyle

Asking for help—See if there are areas he's been struggling with that he couldn't get help for because of his wife's denial.

Service utilization—Determine interest in early-stage AD support groups or similar relevant programs.

Beyond working with these or other goals the man identifies, if time allows you might do or connect him with care management to help the family in additional ways. And, of course, the wife in this case needs support (from you or someone else) to come to terms with her husband's condition.

Case Examples: A Few Last Reflections

These case examples are presented as being in one slice of time, and the length of different readers' counseling interventions will vary by setting and resources. So, how much you can tackle and accomplish within and beyond your sessions gets determined as each individual situation comes along. And, whatever you and your counselees decide to focus on may shift as things continue to happen once you've met them. Perhaps you can see from the foregoing stories how difficult it would be to make progress in multiple areas if you only have eight weeks! And yet, even if that is your constraint, you simply do the best you can in the time available, and know that it will be valued.

You couldn't be expected to know everything about counseling PWESD without some preparation, instruction, and, ultimately, experience. Even then you won't always know, because there is no one right way to respond to these tough circumstances. Rely on your intuition and best judgment and know that those you work with will meet you halfway. Use the framework to delineate, ground, and organize your approach; let it be a beacon for navigating this uncharted territory. Across the case examples presented here we demonstrated the use of all eighteen areas—and we could have interchanged them in countless combinations.

This is just a starting point for training purposes. We can't anticipate together all possible scenarios as they are as infinite as the number of people with early dementia. But you've now glimpsed through the hologram of this fascinating multidimensional undertaking. You've viewed what can come before you through the lens of the PWESD's perspective. And when you establish a relationship with that at its core, you are guaranteed to start witnessing some tales of heroic transformation of your own.

CHAPTER 9

Reaching Out to Find Counseling Participants

Now that the clinical picture of counseling PWESD has been painted, the tale will traverse along the path of program development considerations. This chapter looks at outreach that needs to be done to let people know your service is available so they will come forward to use it. This is not a minor detail! All of your hard work and efforts to fund, develop, educate, and train yourself and other counselors will be most rewarded if you get the word out widely about what you have to offer.

Outreach to recruit people that are appropriate for counseling will probably fall to you or your agency. Even though there is more public awareness about AD than there used to be, for the most part it is not usually about the early stages or the possibility of going on with life. So, we have to craft that message and put it out there—in ways that intrigue and attract people enough to overcome the fear and stigma inherent in identifying with having AD.

You also have to let people within your own work setting and local network know what you are offering. It's very easy for PWESD to otherwise be overlooked by missed opportunities when they themselves call for help, which is happening more and more now. Too, when professionals are aware of your new service, it expands your referral sources and carves your new niche clearly onto the regional continuum of care.

There are a number of ways to do outreach, including seeking publicity through mainstream media; alerting aging and dementia care providers in your community; offering education to the public and professionals in your region; involving PWESD in your agency in various ways; and eliciting culture change within your own organization.

Create Publicity

Counseling for PWESD can be publicized through numerous media formats. A press release aids in contacting newspapers, magazines, and radio stations. In today's world you'll also want to be visible through the Internet and social media. Seek opportunities not only to list or advertise the service but also to relay a more in-depth story. Your article will be even more powerful if it includes an interview with a PWESD. Work closely to educate and monitor reporters if possible so that a positive perspective is conveyed. Attempt to change the language and focus from solely the statistics and horrors of AD to more optimistic phrases about people continuing to function well for some time after being diagnosed in the early stage. You will have to be assertive and persistent to initiate and follow up on this.

On the other hand, the media have come a long way in recent years. There are now more inspirational stories about older people in general. For example, newspapers wrote about Les Paul, the creator of famous guitars, who played music weekly in New York City clubs until he died in his 90s. And, a Japanese woman was written up in a San Francisco newspaper when she became the first woman, and only the fourth person, to achieve judo's highest level—a 10th-degree black belt—at 98 years old! At four foot ten inches and one hundred pounds, she is the granddaughter of a samurai, and her motto is, *"Be strong, be gentle, be beautiful!"* Let me reiterate—neither of these people had dementia. But such complimentary images of aging have not been the norm over the years in mainstream media.

Nowadays we are also more likely to see the media talk about people having AD but courageously admitting it and continuing with their careers for as long as they can. For example, Glen Campbell, who was diagnosed at age 75 after fifty years in the music business, has been profiled in *People* and *Rolling Stone* magazines. After announcing his diagnosis publicly, he released an album and launched a farewell tour before retiring. He still loved what he did, but he didn't want people to think he was drunk onstage if he forgot things while performing.

Similarly, the media's generous coverage of Pat Summitt was quite remarkable. The University of Tennessee college basketball coach, who won more games and national championships than any other coach, was diagnosed with early-onset AD at age 59. She courageously disclosed her diagnosis publicly, remarking that this actually helped her to recover her confidence. She was widely quoted acknowledging that she might have some limitations but intended to keep going as long as possible, and said, *"It is what it is—I've got to face it."* Those close to her said that she displayed the same traits she always had: dedication, perseverance, fierce will, and energy; a sense of centeredness, resolve, and deep inner strength.[1] As Summitt began to need more assistance with coaching over time, she took on less of a central role and eventually retired. But she also became an Alzheimer's advocate, starting a foundation and speaking at related events. Ultimately she received from President Barack Obama the country's highest civilian honor—the Presidential Medal of Freedom. Each of these accomplishments was followed and featured by multiple news sources.

This heartening depiction of a person with dementia is a far cry from the usual stereotypical media messages of the past! It mirrors the whole arc of the counseling process: from accepting the disease to adjusting to it, to finally progressing to further impairment—but all described with respect and reverence. There are many other people in all of our local communities who are perhaps less famous, but no less triumphant, that we can write about in the service of program outreach.

Outreach to the Aging and AD Networks in Your Region

PWESD can be referred to you for counseling through many doorways. They and their families may enter the local service continuum at a variety of points—all of which can then point them toward you. For example, some may already be on a dementia care pathway through an AD diagnostic and research center, a chapter of the Alzheimer's Association, an affiliate of Alzheimer's Foundation of America, or other related organizations. Others may already be in contact with general agencies serving seniors such as area agencies on aging, physicians and other health professionals at medical clinics, neurologists, hospitals, and senior centers. Or, adult children may be connected to family support agencies, adult education settings, employee assistance programs, mental health providers, or psychologists. Families needing help may become obvious to those in religious or other faith communities.

Many providers who come in contact with these folks won't be specialized in early-stage AD and will be glad to know that you are. You can inform them about your new service through phone calls and personal visits, or letters that enclose flyers or brochures for posting and distribution. You can do presentations at staff or aging coalition meetings, Grand Rounds, and conferences. You might have a display booth at health fairs and educational events. Ask agencies to write about the counseling in their newsletters. Let them know the referral process and criteria for participating that we'll be covering in Chapter 10. Be sure to include organizations serving various cultural groups and approach bilingual/bicultural staff for help with spreading the word. Also, call or send letters to your current early-stage clients if you have some attending support groups or other programs or classes you have done.

You want your program description to be clear as well as appealing and hopeful, without promising anything you can't do (like cure the disease). Figure 9.1 shows an example of a postcard used by the grant partners in this project. Figure 9.2 shows another example of possible text for a flyer.

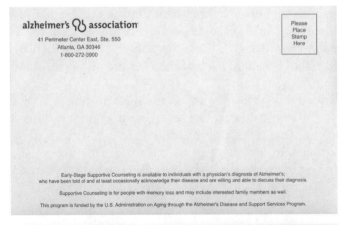

Figure 9.1. Sample outreach postcard (Reprinted by permission of the Alzheimer's Association, Georgia Chapter)

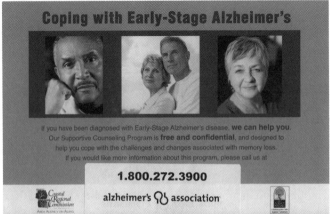

Living Well with Early-Stage Alzheimer's Disease

Counseling is available to help understand and cope with memory loss and related issues. Many people find that a full and meaningful life can continue for some time when they have guidance in adjusting to their condition.

[Trained professionals] are offering education and support to those who have been told they have a physician's diagnosis of early-stage Alzheimer's disease, and are willing and able to talk about it.

Contact us at _____ for more information.

[Agency or provider]

Figure 9.2. Sample outreach flyer

Educate the Public and Professionals in Your Region

Another way to launch your new service is to offer a public education event. You can partner with related agencies, and offer continuing education to professionals. You might provide some very brief, basic information about the disease, but not so much that it replicates other workshops that are generally much more available. Rather, you want to offer something that people may never have seen and heard before. Titles like the following have been successfully used for lectures by this author to help many organizations across the country and around the world "kick off" early-stage support groups:

Learning about and Living with Early-Stage Alzheimer's Disease

Early-Stage Alzheimer's Disease: Focusing on Vitality and Capability

Resilience and Empowerment in the Early Stages of Alzheimer's Disease

A suggested format would begin with introducing the issues that people are uniquely dealing with in the early stages. This can be followed by a PWESD and family member (or two—perhaps different constellations including spouse and adult child) talking about their experiences, and how your agency programs have been helpful—including counseling if they have done it with you. You could have other speakers on various related topics, and breakout sessions for small-group discussions. If you don't have someone who has participated in counseling, you can show a short video with PWESD talking, or illustrate the service with case examples. All of this challenges and refutes the usual stereotypes about AD and gives people a radical first-person view. You'll be letting the public and professionals know who's right for the service and how to access it—all while conveying hope about and putting a positive spin on the disease.

There are many ways to do events like this. Some regions even have entire conferences with only PWESD in the audience. What's suggested here is useful, though, as a starting point for those who don't yet have early-stage services well-known by the community.

Involving PWESD in Your Organization and Events

In the last decade or so, many agencies have taken up the commitment to include people with dementia in their organizations' activities. PWESD are now part of boards, advisory groups, awareness campaigns, public policy efforts, and, as mentioned, public speaking events. Alzheimer's Disease International states that it is the *right* of people with dementia to be involved in representing their own interests:

> The fundamental principle to remember when involving people with dementia is to ask them for their views and listen to what they say. Do not assume that you can

act or speak on their behalf. Involving people with dementia is a new direction for many that with careful planning and support can only help to improve the effectiveness of Alzheimer associations.[2]

In recent years PWESD have given input into how they can best be engaged and supported as speakers, volunteers, research interviewees, and in meetings.[3] There are specific steps that can be taken to facilitate participation, such as preparing for a presentation with clear guidelines. Some people prefer to be interviewed rather than to speak from notes.

Whatever the forum or format, the involvement of PWESD must be handled in a way that is respectful and not exploitative. While it may not have occurred to them, once under way they typically appreciate opportunities to be educators and advocates, and they feel good about doing it. So keep those who are appropriate and available for these activities in mind as a potential resource.

Changing the Culture of Your Organization

Once your agency goes down the road of offering early-stage counseling, it is helpful to integrate the PWESD perspective throughout its entire culture. That is, internally you want to educate all staff, administrators, volunteers, and board members about early-stage issues and the new service. Training anyone who answers the phone or provides assistance to families on how to talk to PWESD directly will help in getting them steered toward you. Externally, you can gear your organization's web site and printed materials toward the PWESD who may be looking for help, and not just their families.

Outreach Is an Intensive Process

Outreach takes a lot of time and energy. In a way, what needs to be done is limitless. On the other hand, whatever you can do goes toward the greater good in terms of raising awareness. The overall idea is that it's advisable to build this into your planning, and to cast a wide net. You will inevitably talk to many PWESD who find out about the counseling but don't meet the criteria to participate, and they will need your time too. In recruiting people to join early-stage support groups, which had similar eligibility guidelines, experience showed that there was an average ratio of 1:4 (i.e., for every four people spoken to, one would be "right" for a group). However, the more we all do these particular types of outreach, the more the information gets out there, and someday it won't take quite as much effort. For now though, it is wise to allow at least a few months for this and the next part of the process.

Referrals to counseling can come from PWESD themselves, their families, or others in their lives, or any number of professionals. If you have done effective outreach, your phone will begin ringing with inquiries. Then you have to be prepared with your screening, selection, and intake protocols. That is what you'll find in the next chapter of the tale.

CHAPTER 10

Assessing and Enrolling Counseling Participants

Now the plot thickens. This is the time to delve more deeply into the process of selecting people who are appropriate for the intervention.

A Multistep Protocol

This is one of the major keys to success in counseling PWESD. Counseling is not beneficial, for example, for those who are in denial about their condition or do not want to talk about it. It is better to find that out before beginning, if possible. However, a certain approach may help to overcome denial, so it's important to give people this opportunity before rushing to judgment.

The process described here affords time over multiple points of contact for people to feel safe in opening up. Telephone screening followed by in-person interviewing involving both PWESD and their families is recommended. These steps will be described, and forms offered for your use. While the protocol may seem long, at the end of it you will be most likely to have people with the right level of ability and willingness to engage in the counseling journey with you. Planning adequate time for this "start-up" activity is all part of building the solid foundation needed to make your new program sustainable.

The selection criteria and procedure laid out here are adapted from those developed by this author for early-stage support groups.[1] They were deemed critical by many colleagues who replicated that program successfully over the years, and are widely used.

Who Should Do the Screening?

Screening allows you to determine the suitability and interest of potential participants and to get their background information. The decision about who is responsible for this depends upon your setting. As a private practitioner, of course, you will do it all. In an agency, the counselor may do it, or others may handle some parts of it. For example, a caseworker might do the intake or even all of the interviewing. Or, a helpline staff person might do the initial telephone prescreening.

There are pros and cons to these different arrangements. The counselor who does all of the initial assessing will have begun a relationship with the PWESD. This is advantageous for starting counseling, where a sense of comfort and trust are so important. The counselor will also be familiar with the PWESD's issues and communication style. While ideal, this will take a lot of the counselor's time; particularly if travel for home visits is involved.

If noncounseling staff are an option for doing the initial assessing, it saves the counselor time. These staff members might also be well able to handle any extra needs that come up, like referrals to other services. The counselor can later review the information gleaned to prepare for working with the PWESD. But the PWESD and counselor will not have met, perhaps requiring more time initially to establish their relationship.

If anyone other than the counselor performs any part of the process described in this chapter, it is most important that the person receive training around talking to people with early dementia. Otherwise, referrals to the counselor are likely to include people who are unsuitable for counseling, such as those who are too impaired. Training can cover the early-stage symptoms, issues, and coping framework, and the need for and benefits of counseling. And, on a more logistical level, how to best integrate this intake and referral process with the agency's usual protocol for enrolling new clients will also need to be determined.

Approaching and Engaging PWESD about Counseling

Chapter 3 on early-stage challenges, Chapter 6 on addressing these challenges, and Chapter 4 on the counseling relationship all talk about the special issue of denial. To summarize, while there is a widespread assumption that most people with dementia are in denial about their condition, this is not true. Some people do hold on to this way of coping, and they would not want or benefit from counseling. Other people are actually quite open to acknowledging their symptoms, and want to learn constructive ways to cope with them. And still others may fluctuate in and out of denial a number of times, or over time. Having the chance and the professional support to work through denial makes a huge difference, and most people have no place to get it. In fact, sometimes what looks like denial is actually a person who was never told (or forgets that they were told) their diagnosis.

In the past, it was widely assumed that PWESD couldn't understand or would react badly to hearing that their diagnosis was AD, and professionals were uncomfortable telling them. Over the years, the consensus has moved more toward the belief that PWESD have a *right* to know their diagnosis just as they would with any other illness.[2] And, a recent report found that growing numbers of families want people with dementia in the early stages to be told.[3] Each situation is different, however, depending on the PWESD's desire to know, the level of insight and cognitive ability, and the family's coping style. In some cases, it might not be right for the person to be told. There is great variability in how this is handled in various medical settings. But the general practice has moved away from people routinely not being told that their diagnosis is AD.

For our purposes here, we need to know that individuals have been told their diagnosis and are cognizant of it to at least some extent. While it can be part of our role to educate them about the disease, it is not our role to be the one to tell them that they have it. This should be done by either a diagnostic or other health professional, or by the family, prior to the person's beginning counseling. If the person who initially calls about counseling is a family member who hasn't discussed the diagnosis with the PWESD, the pros and cons of doing so may be part of what you talk about.

If the PWESD first calls directly about counseling, this is one of the main concerns. Where is this person at on the spectrum of acknowledging that he or she has AD? And how likely is the person to admit this to you or any total stranger on the phone? Because each PWESD is unique, and because each may become willing to talk about the disease at any point in the intake process, there are some things we can do to encourage honest self-disclosure:

- Never force someone to confront or admit his or her impairments. Rather, just continue offering your attention around it.

- Create a climate of respect and acceptance as you develop rapport from the first time you talk with someone. Show that you are a good listener, that you care about the person's opinions and perspectives, and that you value each individual's personhood.

- Use a tone that conveys empathy and that you are not threatening or judgmental.

- Speak with language that reduces defensiveness if that seems like an issue. For example, you can talk about aging, changes in the brain, or memory loss before using the term "AD."

- Demonstrate familiarity with the person's situation. For instance, you can say something like, "*Other people with memory loss sometimes feel frustrated when they lose their train of thought or can't find a word—is this something you ever experience?"*

- Give the person plenty of time to answer you, or to come around to discussing his or her symptoms and concerns. Try more than once in a conversation to gently approach the topic.

- Introduce the counseling from an optimistic and positive standpoint, such as, *"We're starting this new program about coping well with early AD, and we're inviting people like yourself with a lot to offer to be pioneers in helping us get it off the ground."*

- Let the person know that there are also other services available in case other services turn out to be more appropriate.

Even when you are thoroughly prepared for these interactions, people may vacillate from acknowledgment of their condition on the phone to denial in the in-person interview; or from acknowledgment in the interview to denial in the counseling session. For those who are strongly holding on to denial despite your attempts to build rapport and use nonthreatening language, back off, thank them for their time, and end the interview. If, rather, you have gotten over this hump, you can be quite direct in discussing the purpose of the counseling and asking people if they want to engage in it.

Guidelines for Selecting Counseling Participants

Selecting counselees is easier when, in addition to a standard protocol, you have clear and consistent criteria to determine each individual's suitability for counseling. You can have this in mind yourself and also provide it to professionals in your community who are potential referral sources.

What follows here pertains to early-stage Alzheimer's disease. You may additionally choose to work with people with MCI who otherwise meet the criteria, though you will want to explain the distinction between this diagnosis and that of probable AD. There may also be people with causes of progressive, irreversible dementia other than AD (e.g., vascular or Lewy body) that could be appropriate for counseling. Those with frontotemporal dementia can be considered on a case-by-case basis to determine whether, for example, their behavior, facility with language, and level of insight are a good match for counseling. The same principles of positive regard when talking to people with these diagnoses hold, of course, whether or not they turn out to be right for this program.

Here are the questions you will consider and address using the forms that follow:

- Does the person have a physician's diagnosis of probable AD or a related disorder?

- Has the person been told the diagnosis by a professional or family member?

- Does the person at least occasionally acknowledge experiencing memory loss, confusion, or other cognitive impairment?

- Is the impairment mild enough to clearly understand and participate in counseling, as evidenced upon interviewing?

- Does the person have good communication skills, such as the ability to express him/herself, sustain conversation, and comprehend others despite speech or word-finding difficulty?

- Is the person willing and able to discuss feelings, concerns, and experiences related to having AD?

- Is the person interested in receiving information, support, and counseling around living with AD? Can he or she understand the purpose and freely give consent to participate?

- Is there a care partner willing and able to be involved, at least as a liaison and contact person?

- Are there other issues that need to be addressed before counseling can begin (e.g., safety issues, logistical issues, insufficiently or untreated medical or psychiatric conditions)?

It should be noted here that the credentials of each counselor and the needs of each counselee will determine whether concurrent psychiatric conditions warrant involvement by additional clinicians. For example, a psychiatrist may be needed to prescribe and oversee medication for someone who is clinically depressed; or someone who is dealing with post-traumatic stress disorder unrelated to the onset of dementia.

When Is a Person Not Appropriate for Counseling?

There are a variety of reasons that people may be assessed as not right for counseling:

- The person has not been diagnosed with dementia.
- The person has not been told that the diagnosis is dementia.
- The person does not acknowledge the symptoms or condition.
- The person is too impaired by dementia to benefit from counseling.
- The person is not interested in counseling.
- Family members do not want the person to participate in counseling.

The earlier in the intake process that people are screened out, the less awkward it will be for the screener and for those making inquiries. People who are not appropriate can be referred to services that better meet their needs. Counseling is not right for everyone, so part of the staff training to do screening should include familiarity with other resources that can be helpful and available.

A Picture of the Process

Before the story of the various steps of assessment unfolds, Figures 10.1 and 10.2 present a graphic illustration of it. Figure 10.1 shows the process when a PWESD calls about counseling directly. Figure 10.2 charts what happens when a family care partner is the one calling to inquire.

Telephone Prescreening

The idea of prescreening is to determine whether a PWESD meets the basic eligibility criteria to enter counseling. It is a structured way to "cut to the chase" so that you don't go on to do a full intake if it won't be necessary. Figure 10.3 (see page 109) contains five questions that can be asked early on whether an inquiry is received by the counselor or other staff handling incoming calls. This script may not need to be followed verbatim, as long as the conversation is geared toward determining the PWESD's level of understanding, ability, and willingness to discuss what he or she is experiencing.

Time spent in lengthy telephone screening reduces the incidence of unnecessary home or office visits, which engage families (and create paperwork!). It insures that only those who meet the selection criteria go on to be interviewed and enrolled. It also prevents starting counseling with people who are unable to do it, and needing to extricate oneself from that situation. Therefore, it saves time in the long run.

You can think of this as *screening out* as well as screening in potential participants. As you become more experienced, asking these questions early on will come more easily. Remember that your goal is determining appropriateness for this counseling program. You aren't screening for dementia in general, assessing overall health, or coordinating care management issues. There are many other needs within these families, as we know. If addressing them is not part of your designated role, then be prepared to explain your focus and to refer them to other resources or staff whose job it is to help.

It is suggested that you keep a tally of how many people you speak to at this initial inquiry stage, who referred them, how many were screened out and why, and how many went on to be enrolled in the counseling service. These data can be used to demonstrate the ongoing need for this and other services.

Telephone Intake

The bulk of initial screening and intake can be done with a care partner, but it is advisable to also talk to PWESD on the phone (at either of these steps) to see how they respond to the idea of counseling. If the reaction is resistance or confusion, it may indicate that an individual is not a good candidate for counseling. If there is interest and agreement and other conditions seem right, an in-person

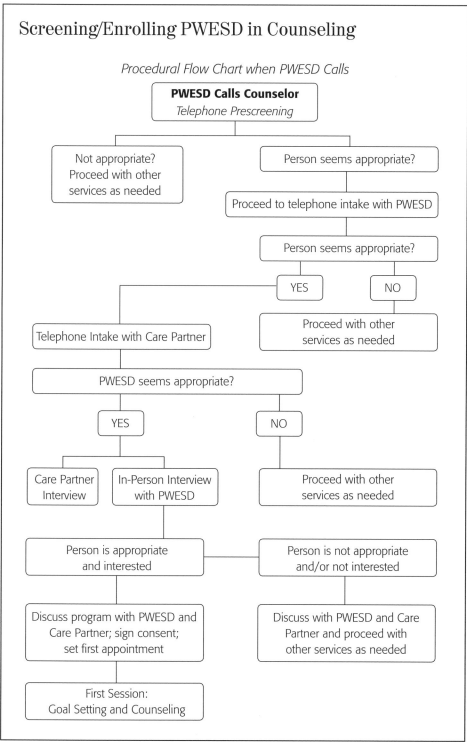

Figure 10.1. Procedural flow chart when PWESD calls to inquire about counseling (Copyright © 2011, by Robyn Yale)

Screening/Enrolling PWESD in Counseling

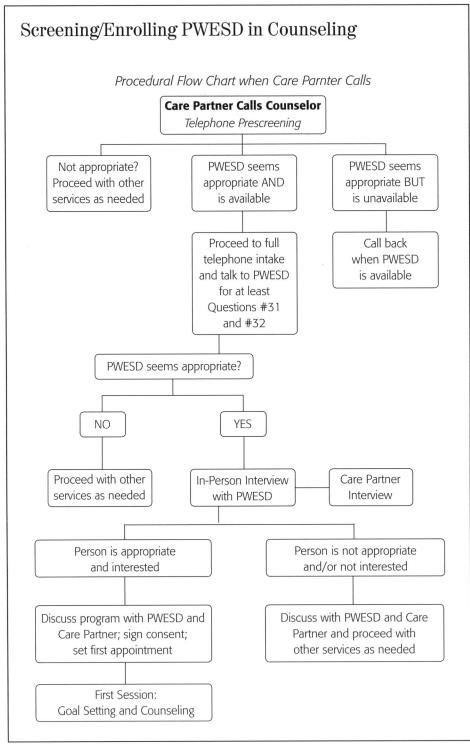

Procedural Flow Chart when Care Parnter Calls

Care Partner Calls Counselor
Telephone Prescreening

Not appropriate? Proceed with other services as needed

PWESD seems appropriate AND is available

PWESD seems appropriate BUT is unavailable

Proceed to full telephone intake and talk to PWESD for at least Questions #31 and #32

Call back when PWESD is available

PWESD seems appropriate?

NO

YES

Proceed with other services as needed

In-Person Interview with PWESD

Care Partner Interview

Person is appropriate and interested

Person is not appropriate and/or not interested

Discuss program with PWESD and Care Partner; sign consent; set first appointment

Discuss with PWESD and Care Partner and proceed with other services as needed

First Session: Goal Setting and Counseling

Figure 10.2. Procedural flow chart when care partner calls to inquire about counseling (Copyright © 2011, by Robyn Yale)

Telephone Prescreening: Five Questions

These questions are directed to the person with early-stage dementia. Parentheses indicate that you are talking instead to a family/care partner rather than the PWESD. Note that this is not really a formal interview, it's meant more to be part of a conversation that gives you an initial sense of the person's suitability for counseling.

1. Are you (or is the person) having any concerns about your memory or daily functioning, for example, forgetting words, trouble managing finances, or anything else?

2. What do you think might be causing these problems? Have you (or has the person) been given any kind of explanation or diagnosis, and if so by whom?

3. How do you feel you are coping with the situation? Do you have family, and how are they coping with the situation? (How do you feel the person is coping with the situation, and how are you as a family member coping?)

4. Have you talked to anyone about your concerns, and if so to whom? (Has the person talked to anyone, and have you?)

5. We have trained professional counselors who provide information and support around living with memory loss. Would you like one of them to call you back to talk further? (Is the person interested in talking to a professional counselor?)

Figure 10.3. Five Questions to Ask in Telephone Prescreening (Copyright © 2011, by Robyn Yale)

---

interview appointment can be made with the care partner's assistance at the end of the intake.

If the initial inquiry call comes directly from a PWESD, and the prescreening questions listed earlier have not already been asked of that person, you have the option of beginning this conversation with these. Again, if conditions seem right you can proceed with the intake, but you are likely to need the care partner's help to get some of the background information on the form. In this case, let the PWESD know that also talking to a care partner is a standard part of the enrollment process.

It is important to clarify for the PWESD and family that the counseling service is primarily for the person with dementia, although family may participate to a limited extent. This will be explained more formally at the end of the enrollment process.

If you are doing the intake with the care partner, you will see that questions 31 and 32 on the following form (Figure 10.4) have you ask to speak to the PWESD. (Here you could use the five prescreening questions listed earlier if you haven't already done so and they would be helpful.) At a minimum, you want to

Telephone Intake

Date __/__/__ Staff person _____

Person with early-stage dementia (PWESD) _____

1. Contact person is a:

   1. PWESD _____

   2. Care partner _____

   3. Professional _____

   4. Other: _____

2. Relationship to PWESD:

   1. Self _____

   2. Relative (Specify: _____)_____

   3. Professional—e.g., caseworker, therapist, etc.

   (Specify:_____) _____

   4. Other: _____

3A. List this contact person's name, address, and phone:

_____

_____

_____

_____

3B. If different, list ongoing contact person's name, address, and phone:

_____

_____

_____

_____

Relationship to PWESD_____

(continued)

Figure 10.4. Telephone Intake (Copyright © 2011, by Robyn Yale)

4. Source of referral:

   1. Family

   2. Friend

   3. Agency or professional (Name _____

                    Phone _____)

   4. Media or other publicity

   (Specify:_____)

   5. Other: _____

5. Information about PWESD:

   Name_____

   Address _____

   _____ Phone _____

6A. When were symptoms of confusion/memory loss first noticed? _____

   _____ Month/Year

6B. When were these symptoms first evaluated? _____

   _____ Month/Year

6C. When were symptoms most recently evaluated? _____

   _____ Month/Year

6D. What was the diagnosis/es?_____

7A. Who determined this diagnosis?

   Name_____ Phone_____

7B. List PWESD's primary physician, if different:

   Name_____

   Address _____

   _____Phone _____

8A. Was PWESD informed of diagnosis?

   1. Y

   2. N   *(continued)*

Figure 10.4.   Telephone Intake (continued)

8B. Who informed PWESD of diagnosis?

   1. MD or other clinicians

   2. Family (Who?:_____)

   3. Other (List: _____)

COMMENTS: _____

_____

_____

8C. When was PWESD informed of diagnosis? _____

_____ Month/Year

9A. What was PWESD told about the diagnosis?

_____

_____

9B. Does PWESD discuss the diagnosis/illness much?

   1. Y

   2. N

9C. What kinds of things does s/he say about it?

_____

_____

10A. Is PWESD able to clearly communicate thoughts?

   1. Y

   2. N

10B. Are there any speech or comprehension problems?

   1. Y

   2. N

DESCRIBE: _____

_____

_____

(continued)

Figure 10.4. Telephone Intake (continued)

10C. Can PWESD tell you how s/he feels?

   1. Y

   2. N

COMMENTS: _____

_____

_____

11A. Does PWESD generally do well in social situations?

   1. Y

   2. N

COMMENTS: _____

_____

_____

11B. What social activities is PWESD currently involved in?

_____

_____

12A. Does PWESD have any other major medical diagnoses?

   1. Y

   2. N

LIST: _____

_____

_____

12B. Has PWESD had any problems for which s/he has seen a psychiatrist?

   1. Y

   2. N

LIST: _____

_____

_____

(continued)

Figure 10.4. Telephone Intake (continued)

12C. Is PWESD currently in therapy?

   1. Y [**TYPE:** ___ Individual ____ Family____ Group____Other]

   2. N

NAME OF CLINICIAN: _____

12D. Is PWESD currently taking any medications?

   1. Y

   2. N

LIST ALL MEDICATIONS:_____

_____

_____

_____

12E. In your opinion, does PWESD overuse alcohol or medications?

   1. Y

   2. N

EXPLAIN: _____

_____

_____

13. Describe any current concerns about PWESD's mood:

   1. Anxiety

   2. Depression

   3. Delusions

   4. Other (List: _____)

   5. None: _____

COMMENTS: _____

_____

_____

(continued)

Figure 10.4.   Telephone Intake (continued)

14. Are there any current behavior problems, such as:

   1. Combativeness

   2. Wandering

   3. Agitation

   4. Other (List: _____)

   5. None: _____

COMMENTS: _____
_____
_____

15. Could PWESD sit through 1-hour counseling sessions without bowel/bladder accidents?

   1. Y

   2. N

16. Do you think PWESD can sit in 1-hour counseling sessions and remain interested?

   1. Y

   2. N

17. Do you think PWESD can understand our explanation of the counseling and sign consent to participate?

   1. Y

   2. N

18. Is PWESD ambulatory?

   1. Ambulates independently

   2. Ambulates with assistance of another person

   3. Ambulates with assistive device

   4. Needs a wheelchair

19. How will PWESD get to counseling sessions? _____
_____

(continued)

Figure 10.4.   Telephone Intake (continued)

20. What is PWESD's age?_____

21. What is PWESD's gender?

    1. M

    2. F

22. What is PWESD's education level?

    1. Less than high school

    2. High school grad

    3. Some college

    4. College graduate

    5. Postgraduate/Professional

23. What is PWESD's race or ethnic group?

    1. American Indian/Alaskan native

    2. Asian/Pacific Islander

    3. African-American

    4. Hispanic

    5. White

    6. Other (List: _____)

_____

PLACE OF BIRTH:_____

PRIMARY ENGLISH-SPEAKING? ___ Y ___ N

24. What is PWESD's living arrangement?

    1. Home, alone

    2. Home, with spouse and/or other relatives

    3. Home, w/nonrelatives

    4. Residential/Board and Care

    5. Other (List: _____)

_____

(continued)

Figure 10.4.   Telephone Intake (continued)

INFORMATION ABOUT CARE PARTNER:

_____

_____

_____

_____

25A. Is care partner willing to be interviewed and be an ongoing contact person?

   1. Y

   2. N

25B. Did care partner know PWESD before memory problem began?

   1. Y

   2. N

LENGTH OF RELATIONSHIP: _____

25C. How often does care partner have contact with PWESD?

   1. Daily

   2. Several times a week

   3. Weekly

   4. Several times a month

   5. Monthly

TYPE OF CONTACT: _____

26. What is care partner's age? _____

27. What is care partner's gender?

   1. M

   2. F

(continued)

Figure 10.4. Telephone Intake (continued)

28. What is care partner's race or ethnic background?
    1. American Indian/Alaskan native
    2. Asian/Pacific Islander
    3. African-American
    4. Hispanic
    5. White
    6. Other (List: ______________________________)

____

PRIMARY ENGLISH-SPEAKING? ___ Y ___N

29. Is care partner employed?
    1. Full time
    2. Part time
    3. Not employed

30. How does care partner rate his/her own health status?
    1. Excellent
    2. Good
    3. Fair
    4. Poor

DETERMINING WHETHER TO INTERVIEW: Ask to speak to PWESD. Ask "Five Telephone Prescreening Questions" (see Figure 10.3) if you haven't already, or otherwise converse to assess willingness, ability, and interest in counseling. Then proceed to answer the following questions:

31. What is PWESD's response (on phone) to the idea of being in counseling?

____

____

32. Does PWESD agree (on phone) to meet for an interview?
    1. Y
    2. N

(continued)

In Yale (2013), *Counseling People with Early-Stage Alzheimer's Disease: A Powerful Process of Transformation.* Health Professions Press, Inc.

Figure 10.4. Telephone Intake (continued)

33A. If PWESD doesn't meet screening criteria, note reason:

_____

_____

_____

33B. If PWESD meets screening criteria but can't otherwise participate in counseling, note reason:

_____

_____

_____

34. Preference for location of counseling appointments_____

35. Preference for time of counseling appointments _____

36. Interview Appointment: Date _____ Time _____

Place _____

SPECIAL NOTES:_____

_____

_____

_____

_____

_____

_____

_____

_____

_____

_____

_____

_____

_____

_____

_____

(end)

Figure 10.4. Telephone Intake (continued)

ascertain comprehension and interest and get the PWESD's permission to set up an in-person interview. You can say something like, *"I've been talking with your (wife, son, etc.) about this program to help people cope with memory loss and s/he thought it might interest you. It involves meeting with a counselor about the challenges and successes you may be experiencing in dealing with this. How does it sound to you?"* The person has an opportunity to express interest, decline, ask questions about the program, or indicate that he or she doesn't understand. If you determine that the person isn't following you or isn't interested and you've tried some of the strategies for engaging PWESD suggested previously, you can thank the individual for the time spent and ask to again speak with the care partner to discuss this reaction.

If someone spoke to the PWESD directly at prescreening and he or she responded favorably to the idea of counseling, but now there is denial or resistance, you can say: *"You spoke to someone here at our agency on the phone and at that time you said you were concerned about your memory and would like a call back in regard to counseling. You may not remember this and that's okay; those kinds of memory slips are exactly what we help people with here."*—and see where that takes you.

The telephone intake form begins on page 110.

In-Person PWESD Interview

If the screening and intake conversations have all been favorable, you can proceed to the next step. The in-person interview begins with the counselor introducing him/herself to the PWESD and care partner together and describing more about the counseling program. The PWESD is then interviewed alone, with the explanation that you are trying to learn about what he or she is experiencing. The individual can be reassured that this is not a "test" and therefore there are no "right answers."

If you preview the interview questions in Figure 10.6, you will see that they'll paint a picture for you of PWESDs' views of their lives, and of their capability of conversing with you. Remember also that all individuals will be different in terms of their readiness to talk about their condition. If you feel you need practice before embarking on an interview like this, you can do the training exercise suggested in Figure 10.5. You will need a colleague or other second person to do it with you.

At question #23 of the PWESD interview in Figure 10.6 (see page 122), the counselor has the option of doing the Mini-Mental Status Exam[4] or the Mini-Cog[5] if there is still uncertainty about the person's cognitive abilities. These are standardized tools widely used to briefly screen for cognitive impairment. You can preface this by saying that you understand the person has already done a lot of testing, but it is a routine part of your interview process and gives you an idea of memory functioning. Most people do not mind doing it. For the early-stage support groups, a score of 18 on the Mini-Mental was used as a general cutoff point. However, please note that these screening tools are just a guideline to supplement your clinical impression; they aren't meant to be the whole basis of your determination. Staff who are going to use either of them should be trained in administering them, although they are not difficult to use.

Two people will role-play the beginning of the PWESD interview three times. They can keep the same roles or switch each time. The purpose is to get a sense of what it's like to talk about these issues. It also demonstrates the variability in self-disclosure, and thus, appropriateness for counseling.

The first time, one person is the counselor and the other is the PWESD. Go through Questions #1–9 of the interview below (see Figure 10.6), and have the PWESD be someone who is very open, cooperative, and forthcoming in the answers. This demonstrates a person who should be easy to interview!

The second time, begin again, going back through the same questions. Now, have the PWESD be completely in denial. The counselor can use approaches discussed previously to see if the resistance lessens, but the PWESD stays in the same place. If you've tried everything that's comfortable for you with no change in response, then this actually illustrates someone who shouldn't have gotten this far in the selection process! (Unless, perhaps, they weren't in denial at the point of screening and/or intake).

The third time, once again go back through the same questions. This time the PWESD starts out denying any problems, but then responds to the counselor by coming to admit some concerns. With a person like this, the interview can proceed—and a relationship has begun.

Figure 10.5. Training Exercise for In-Person PWESD Interview (Copyright © 2011, by Robyn Yale)

Upon completion of the in-person PWESD interview here, one could also incorporate additional scales of concern, such as one for mood or other outcome measures that are being pre- and post-tested.

Care Partner Interview

The role of family in this counseling program was discussed in Chapter 7. It is recommended that you interview the care partner even if he or she will only be minimally involved in the counseling (Figure 10.7). This can help to verify the self-report from the PWESD interview, give you a sense of the family's perspective and needs, and put the care partner at ease in getting to know you.

If you happen to have the luxury of two staff persons available, the care partner can be interviewed at the same time as the PWESD. Otherwise, this can happen afterward, or even on the phone.

You may want to modify or adapt the care partner interview form (see page 128) if, for example, you are doing research, individual counseling with family members, or more intensive joint counseling with PWESD and care partners than this book covers.

Person with Early-Stage Dementia In-Person Interview

Date __/__/__ Staff person _____ PWESD Name _____

1. What, if any, problems are you having with confusion or memory loss?

2. I'll now go through a few of the areas that may or may not be difficult for you. Do you have any trouble mixing up:

    1. Times of the day or days

    2. People

    3. Places you find yourself

    4. None of the above

COMMENTS: _____
    _____
    _____

3. Do you have difficulty with things like:

    1. Finding the right words, or recalling words or names

    2. Reading, or recalling some things you read

    3. Managing your own or your household finances

    4. Driving

    5. None of the above

COMMENTS: _____
    _____
    _____

(continued)

Figure 10.6. Person with Early-Stage Dementia In-Person Interview (Copyright © 2011, by Robyn Yale)

4. Are there any other areas we haven't discussed that are troublesome for you?

5. What do you think is the cause of these difficulties you've been having?

6. Have you been told anything by a doctor or anyone else about the cause or diagnosis of these problems? If so, what?

7A. Have you tried to get more information about your condition, for example, from medical professionals, agencies, family members, or books?

(continued)

Figure 10.6.   PWESD In-Person Interview (continued)

7B. Is there any particular information you would like to get?

8. Do you usually talk to anyone about your diagnosis or the problems you've been having? If so, whom?

9. Is there anyone else you'd like to talk to about the problems you've been having? If so, whom?

10. Think back to before these problems began. How has your life changed since you first noticed that you had a problem?

(continued)

Figure 10.6. PWESD In-Person Interview (continued)

11. I'd like to ask about how you spend your time now. Are you doing any paid or volunteer work?

12. Were you previously involved in paid or volunteer work?

13. What types of hobbies, interests, leisure activities are you doing now?

14. Are there any hobbies or activities you did in the past that you aren't doing anymore?

15. Tell me about your social life. Do you:

   1. Belong to clubs

   2. Go to church or other religious functions

   3. See friends regularly

   4. Other (specify)

COMMENTS: _____

_____

_____

(continued)

Figure 10.6. PWESD In-Person Interview (continued)

16. Who are the people closest to you?

    1. Spouse

    2. Children

    3. Other relatives (who?)

    4. Friends

    5. Other (specify)

17. Is there any way in which your relationships with (people identified) have changed?

18. If it seems to you that overall your life has changed somewhat, how do you feel about this?

19. How would you say you've been feeling in general?

(continued)

Figure 10.6. PWESD In-Person Interview (continued)

20. How would you say that your mood has been over the past month? (e.g., cheerful, sad, irritable, etc.)

21. Do you worry much? If so, what kinds of things do you worry about?

22. I'm here today to offer you counseling around the challenges and successes of living with memory loss. Have you ever been in counseling before? If yes, how was it for you?

23. Now I need to do some short testing of your memory and then we'll be finished.

    MMSE or Mini-Cog SCORE:_____

    Thank you for your patience and cooperation!

Staff Observations/Notes: (insight, communication, orientation, family interaction, etc.):

(end)

Figure 10.6. PWESD In-Person Interview (continued)

Care Partner (CP) Interview

Date __/__/__ Staff person _____ CP Name_____

1. What kinds of things do you regularly need to assist PWESD with, in terms of self-care or other activities of daily living?

2. Do you find that you deal with any specific problematic behaviors (e.g., PWESD repeating questions or following you around)?

3. Can you give some examples of your relative's cognitive difficulties (e.g., word-finding, not understanding things you explain)?

4. Does PWESD ever talk with you about the problems s/he has been having? If so, what does s/he say?

(continued)

Figure 10.7. Care Partner Interview (Copyright © 2011, by Robyn Yale)

5. What does PWESD think is the cause of these problems?

6. What was PWESD told about the diagnosis of these problems, and by whom?

7. Does PWESD talk to anyone else about the diagnosis or the problems s/he has been having? If so, to whom?

8. Has PWESD tried to get more information about the problems s/he has been having? If so, from where?

9. Think back to before these problems began. How has PWESD's life changed since the time these problems began?

(continued)

Figure 10.7.   Care Partner Interview (continued)

10. Is PWESD currently doing any paid or volunteer work?

11. How is this a change from PWESD's previous work life?

    1. Change in responsibilities

    2. Works fewer hours

    3. Stopped working

    4. Started new type of work

    5. Other (specify)

12. What types of hobbies, interests, leisure activities does PWESD do now?

13. Are there any hobbies or activities s/he did in the past that s/he doesn't do anymore?

(continued)

Figure 10.7.   Care Partner Interview (continued)

14. Tell me about PWESD's social life. Does s/he:

   1. Belong to clubs

   2. Go to church or other religious functions

   3. See friends regularly

   4. Other (specify:)

COMMENTS: _____

_____

_____

15. Are there ways in which PWESD's social life has changed since the onset of the illness?

16. Who are the people closest to PWESD?

   1. Spouse

   2. Children

   3. Other relatives (who?)

   4. Friends

   5. Other (specify)

17. Is there any way in which PWESD's relationships with (people identified) have changed?

(continued)

Figure 10.7.   Care Partner Interview (continued)

18. Are there ways in which things at home have changed (e.g., PWESD who used to manage finances no longer does so)?

19. Has PWESD completed a:
    1. Power of attorney for health care
    2. Power of attorney for finances
    3. Both of the above
    4. Neither of the above

20. Are there any changes we haven't discussed that are troublesome for PWESD?

21. If it seems to you that PWESD's life has changed, how do you think s/he feels about this?

22. How would you say PWESD's mood has been in the past month?

(continued)

Figure 10.7.   Care Partner Interview (continued)

23. Do moods change frequently or extremely? If yes, please describe.

24. Does PWESD worry much? If so, about what kinds of things?

25. Are there any changes we haven't discussed that are troublesome for you as a care partner?

26. In general, how would you say you are managing with the care partner responsibilities?

27. Do you have concerns about your own mood or stress level?

(continued)

Figure 10.7.   Care Partner Interview (continued)

28. Have you yourself sought more information about your relative's illness? If so, from where?

29. Have you used any community services, such as care partner support groups, day or in-home respite care, counseling, etc.?

30. Would you like information on these or other services?

31. I'm here today to offer counseling to PWESD around the challenges and successes of living with memory loss. Has s/he ever been in counseling before? If so, how did it work out?

(continued)

Figure 10.7.   Care Partner Interview (continued)

32. In your view, what might be important emotional, practical, or lifestyle goals for PWESD to work on? (give some examples)

33. Where will you be during group sessions?

34. List name, address, and phone of person(s) to contact in case of emergency:

Thank you for your patience and cooperation!

Staff Observations/Notes: (care partner's view of symptoms, care partner functioning, family interaction, etc.):

(end)

Figure 10.7.   Care Partner Interview (continued)

Some PWESD do not have a care partner that is willing or able to participate in counseling. It is preferable, however, to at the very least have someone in the role of liaison for things like offering background information, helping to set and maintain appointments, and providing transportation to sessions. It may be possible to find a friend, neighbor, or involved professional to act as a contact person when there is no family available.

Enrollment Agreement/Consent Form

If the interview has confirmed your impression that the PWESD is a good candidate for counseling, you may want to have an enrollment agreement signed, like that in Figure 10.8. While not legally binding, it establishes the understanding that certain expectations have been communicated. Again, you may choose to modify the basic sample given here. For example, if families will be more prominently involved, the wording can be altered to reflect that. If you are doing research, different language will be required by your institutional review board for consent to participate. Other agencies could have the document reviewed by an attorney to incorporate a waiver of liability. Chances are that this formality won't be called upon, but some may like to have it included.

This stage of the process also gives you an opportunity to explain the boundaries of confidentiality, as discussed earlier. And, here you can reiterate the terms under which counseling might end, as covered in Chapter 4. If you decide to use a written agreement along the lines of the example presented in Figure 10.8, both the PWESD and the care partner should receive a copy of it.

Conclusion: Selection/Enrollment Process

While it may be tempting to circumvent the screening, selection, and enrollment processes, it is strongly suggested that you do them. Though lengthy, the forms are thorough, and each has a purpose that gives you valuable information. Though they take your time to do, these steps can also save you as well as families time and potential embarrassment.

In the pilot project you will soon read about, one counselor in training said that she learned a lesson when she didn't follow the recommended protocol. She spoke extensively to a husband on the phone whose wife with dementia was not available at the time. The counselor then invited the couple in for the next step of interviewing, and discovered immediately that the wife was further along than early-stage, and was also not interested in counseling. It became clear that the husband either didn't understand the parameters of the program, or was not able to acknowledge the extent of his wife's impairment (or perhaps both). The counselor then saw why talking to the person with dementia on the phone at the intake stage is necessary, and found it comfortable to do so thereafter.

Early-Stage Dementia Counseling Program Enrollment/Consent Form

This agreement invites you to participate in a new counseling program. Sessions will be held with and focused on the needs of the person with early-stage dementia. Care partners may be involved to some extent, depending upon the direction taken. The emphasis will be on identifying the concerns and challenges that come with having dementia, and developing ways to cope effectively with those challenges. Care partners are welcome to call (name of agency or counselor) for information about additional services that are available to them.

A trained counselor will provide (number of, or ongoing) weekly counseling sessions for the person with early-stage dementia. Each meeting will last about one hour. When counseling ends, you will be asked to complete a short survey about your participation to help us evaluate the program.

It is recommended that the care partner plan to transport the person with early-stage dementia to and from any counseling sessions that do not take place at the person's home. If you have a different plan for transportation, please state it here:

_____

_____

_____

The specific content of counseling sessions is considered confidential and will not be shared with care partners without the person with dementia's permission, unless such concerns arise as a health or safety emergency. General information about the counselee's progress will be conveyed to care partners as appropriate. Counselors do have the legal responsibility to report suspected cases of abuse, neglect, or exploitation—or any serious threat to harm self or others—to the proper authorities.

The costs to you for participating in this program will be (none, fee, sliding scale, etc). Payment will be scheduled (how/when).

Counseling can continue as long as the person with dementia remains aware of and acknowledges his/her condition; is able to fully participate; and wants to be doing it. The counselor will raise any concerns about a change in status to the person and family as soon as it is noticed, giving as much time as possible to determine whether to continue. If counseling needs to end, every effort will be made to help the person with dementia and care partner transition smoothly to other services.

(continued)

In Yale (2013), *Counseling People with Early-Stage Alzheimer's Disease: A Powerful Process of Transformation.* Health Professions Press, Inc. All rights reserved.

Figure 10.8. Sample Enrollment Agreement/Consent Form (Copyright © 2011, by Robyn Yale)

I have read or had read to me the description of the Early-Stage Dementia Counseling Program and would like to enroll in it.

_____

Signature of Primary Participant   Date _____

I have read this agreement and will serve as a contact person for the counselor.

_____

Signature of Care Partner   Date _____

_____

Signature of Person Conducting Interview   Date _____

Figure 10.8.   Sample Enrollment Agreement/Consent Form (continued)

Once you become more familiar with the procedure, the population, and your own assessment skills you may consider consolidating these various forms. And, if you already know the counselee from other contact or programs, streamlining the interviewing might naturally occur. As mentioned, the forms can also be adapted for the aims of different practice or research settings. The bottom line is that we have a way to discern who can best engage in counseling. And, we demonstrate from the start of our contact with families that the PWESD is at the table and central to the team.

Finally, it's important to say that there are no forms that override clinical judgment. This is the essence of the human element, and will guide you throughout your work with these clients. The forms provide a system, but it's best to trust your own intuition first and foremost.

CHAPTER 11

Evaluating Counseling and Progress Toward Goals

Counseling Begins with Goal Setting

After all of the assessment and enrollment paperwork just explained is completed, the first session of counseling begins with setting goals for your work together. In Chapter 5, we walked through this initial process. Goals reflect the emotional, practical, and lifestyle challenges that PWESD encounter, and can organize and prioritize each individual's unique concerns. The inspiration for the form used in that section and again in this one will be more fully identified when the results of the pilot project are presented in Chapter 13. The form serves as a guide to the Framework for Coping with Early Dementia; a structure for counseling efforts; a means of later reviewing progress toward goals; a potential baseline for outcome measures if they are used; and a tool for evaluation of the counselor and program.

Evaluation of Progress Toward Goals

The current of our story now carries us to the time that counseling ends. Here we want to explore how far the person feels he or she has come in working on the goals that were set. We also benefit from feedback about the counselor and counseling sessions.

Figure 11.1 provides a means to evaluate progress toward counseling goals, which can be conducted through a conversation. The PWESD gets a copy, and together you review the areas of concern selected as well as any additional ones that were impacted. Depending on the length of your time together, the gauge may be that people feel they've begun to work toward certain things (e.g., accepting their condition, or completing powers of attorney) rather than finished accomplishing them.

Evaluation of Counseling

Following this, Figure 11.1 has some open-ended questions to garner comments about the counseling experience. If you are a private practitioner, this can be done in a less formal way. If you are in an agency that needs program evaluation data, it might be important to obtain the feedback without the counselor present. In some cases, the PWESD may be able to fill it out as a written questionnaire. If the person is unable to do so alone, though, family or other staff (if available) can assist. Alternatively, other staff can do a verbal interview. However, since that person is not familiar, the PWESD's sense of continuity and comfort may be affected. Still, this has the overall advantage of being a more objective and unbiased process.

Additional Sources of Data

Depending on your time, interest, and mandates, it is possible to measure the results of counseling in other, broader ways.

Outcome Research

If you are doing research, you'll need some additional measures of success. Tying the achievement of distinct goals to a change in well-being and other areas would require more rigorous design and investigation of cause and effect. A very specific protocol for interviewing PWESD would be required, too.

Those who have the skills and resources are encouraged to further refine and standardize instruments that can yield quantifiable results specific and sensitive to early dementia. Validated scales in such areas as mood and self-esteem can be used before and after counseling to assess the effect of this approach. Development of a measure that captures coping with the emotional, practical, and lifestyle issues faced in early AD would be an invaluable addition to this and other psychosocial intervention studies.

Counseling Sessions

Documenting the themes and interactions that occur in counseling sessions provides a record to use (generally, respecting confidentiality) for reports, education,

Evaluating Early-Stage Alzheimer's Disease Counseling

	Made Progress	Was Already Addressing	Wasn't a Concern
Emotional Adjustment:			
Understanding, acknowledging, and becoming more accepting of my condition			
Working toward finding new meaning/purpose in life			
Redefining my identity and feeling good about who I am			
Expressing feelings (both positive and negative) about my situation			
Having an attitude of being strong and capable			
Letting other people know that I want to be treated with respect			
Practical Coping Strategies:			
Learning and using stress management techniques			
Using memory aids and strategies			
Enhancing my ability to communicate, and informing others about it			
Paying more attention to physical exercise, diet, rest, and general health			
Doing memory and other cognitive exercise activities			
Getting emotional support from others			
Lifestyle Issues:			
Doing and/or developing new social and vocational activities			

(continued)

Figure 11.1. Evaluating Early-Stage Alzheimer's Disease Counseling (Copyright © 2011, by Robyn Yale)

	Made Progress	Was Already Addressing	Wasn't a Concern
Talking about and making future legal, financial, health, and care planning decisions			
Acknowledging and working on challenges and changes with my family			
Asking for and accepting help from others			
Using early-stage support services			
Taking steps to problem-solve safety issues such as driving or managing finances			

TOP GOAL PRIORITIES_____

_____

_____

Please describe how you feel you've made (or haven't made) progress in these areas

_____

_____

Additional Goals _____

_____

_____

Please describe how you feel you've made progress in these areas _____

_____

_____

Do you feel that counseling improved your ability to understand and cope with your condition? _____

_____

_____

(continued)

Figure 11.1.   Evaluating Early-Stage Alzheimer's Disease Counseling (continued)

What did you find helpful about the counseling?_____

_____

_____

Was there anything that was not helpful about the counseling? _____

_____

_____

Is there anything you would suggest changing about the counseling process? _____

_____

_____

Do you have any comments about the time, place, length, or amount of counseling?

_____

_____

Would you like to continue counseling? _____

_____

_____

Do you have any comments about the counselor?_____

_____

_____

Any other comments?_____

_____

_____

(end)

Figure 11.1. Evaluating Early-Stage Alzheimer's Disease Counseling (continued)

funding, and project justification. The variability in each person's situation and the range of possible reactions are fascinating, and we are all still learning how we can best assist. Keeping case notes captures the issues that come up, key aspects of the therapeutic alliance, and other highlights of this interesting and intimate relationship.

Perceptions of the Family/Care Partner

The previous chapter on enrolling participants included a form for interviewing families about PWESD's concerns as well as their own. If you are offering separate or joint counseling to care partners then you would want to have them evaluate their progress and the counseling at the end as well. You might also design questions that get at changes in the family system as a result of the intervention.

In the model presented in this book, the person with dementia is the primary counselee, and families are only peripherally involved. Still, it's illuminating to ask about their perceptions of how the PWESD responded to the intervention. You might inquire along these lines:

- Do you think counseling was helpful to the PWESD, and if so, how?

- If you don't think counseling was helpful, why not?

- Do you have any concerns about the PWESD's reaction to counseling?

- Did you notice any effect of counseling on the PWESD, such as change in mood, behavior, or action after counseling sessions?

- What did the PWESD say about counseling?

- Has the PWESD's counseling affected you or your family in any way?

- Do you have any comments about the counselor?

- Do you have any suggestions for changes to the counseling that was provided?

- Any other comments?

The Counselor's Experience

The person with the bird's-eye view of whether the counseling helped PWESD feel and cope better with early dementia is, of course, the counselor. And, many counselors will be newly practicing with this population, since the service is not widely available now. It can be enlightening for counselors in private practice to reflect on the following questions, or for counselors in agencies to provide feedback on them:

- Do you feel counseling was helpful to PWESD? How/why?

- Are there any ways in which you feel that counseling was not helpful?

- Do you have any suggestions for changes to the counseling protocol that you used?

- Are there any ways in which you feel counseling was helpful or not helpful to care partners?

- What learning needs or concerns did you have initially? (e.g., how to talk to someone about having dementia; how to know who is right for counseling, how to answer difficult questions about AD, etc.)

- Do you have a better understanding of these areas now?

- Were there benefits to you personally and/or professionally from the counseling experience? (e.g., personal growth, professional competence, etc.)

- Did this program have any effect on your agency? (e.g., referrals, staff expertise, service utilization, etc.)

- Do you feel that there were any benefits to the local service community from having this counseling available?

Evaluation: Summary

Evaluation tells us about the impact of counseling on increasing PWESD's coping abilities. We also gain valuable information about the structure, format, and techniques we employ. We can apply what we are told to many activities: modifying and strengthening counseling skills; providing reports to funders and administrative auspices; and documenting service needs and effectiveness for training, program development, and advocacy purposes.

CHAPTER 12

A Segue Sideways

A Few Other Considerations

The tale's previous three chapters covered some administrative aspects of this counseling model. And Chapters 4 and 5 talked about counseling from a clinical vantage point. Here are a few logistical and other odds and ends that didn't easily fold into those sections but are also important to consider.

Where Should Counseling Take Place?

There are a few options for where counseling (and initial screening/enrollment, and evaluation) can take place. It might work best for you to have people come to your office. Ideally you would want them to be brought there and back home by someone else, rather than wonder if they will be able to find their way alone. At the very least, you want to know how to contact someone else at those times in case there is a problem.

However, coming to the office may be hard for some people if they don't drive or if the distance is great. Having counseling in people's homes provides them with the familiarity and comfort of their own environment. But, the home needs to be conducive in terms of privacy and the ability to concentrate without distractions or interruptions. There needs to be an understanding with care partners around whether or not they will be involved in any part of the meeting, and where they will be otherwise.

While having the counselor do home visits may be most convenient for PWESD and their families, the costs in terms of time, fuel, and pressure for the counselor need to be factored into program development.

Finally, in this day and age some counselors work over the Internet or via Skype. These mediums would not work as well for people with dementia, who could have trouble with technology as well as with tracking and recognition. The counselor's nuanced perceptions might also be impeded. And, these techniques do not optimize the personal, human connection that is so critical for this particular intervention.

When Should Sessions Be Scheduled?

It's recommended that counseling sessions be set for late morning or early afternoon, as generally speaking, these are the best times for PWESD. Of course, you need to check this out with each person. You have to work around their schedules, and can't make assumptions. For example, while one counselor in the pilot project kept coming up against her client's medical appointments, another's client was quite busy practicing for her flash mob! (You just never know . . . !)

Calling to remind the person prior to the meeting time is a good practice, since forgetting can obviously occur.

How Long Should Sessions Be?

Sessions have been held for forty-five minutes, an hour, or sixty to ninety minutes. You can either have a set time for everyone, or vary it with each person's ability and your own time frame. In either case, you want to be clear about your maximum session length, and stick to ending at that point. You may also end sooner if a PWESD seems ready to do that.

How Many Sessions Should There Be?

The number of counseling sessions is determined by multiple factors. The pilot project on which this book was based created an eight-week model, primarily because funding was limited by a one-time grant. There is no magic about the reason for eight weeks over ten, twelve, or any other number in and of itself. The model is adaptable, and you can decide how to use it depending upon your available resources.

In fact, a period like eight weeks is extremely short for individuals coming to terms with having dementia, implementing new coping strategies, and in many cases giving up huge parts of their life or identity. Yet, eight weeks if it's all you have can certainly still be valuable. You just have to be realistic about what you can accomplish. Offering what you can is an improvement over no individual attention at all. The counseling relationship has the potential to catalyze processes of accepting, adjusting, and problem-solving that might not otherwise be possible.

Ideally, counseling would be offered for as long as it can be helpful. Chapter 8 gives a personal example of working with someone for over a year. This allows you to deal with the ongoing nature of challenges and changes that occur. The luxury of time affords PWESD opportunities to not only see what is necessary but to take action, and then for the two of you to navigate the next impending cascades.

Chapter 4 talked about ending counseling under the different scenarios of time-limited or longer-term intervention. Counselees need to understand how the determination to end counseling will be made and when that will happen. If possible, they should be central to the decision, and have plenty of notice when it's being considered or is structured to happen. This is likely to represent yet another loss, so must be handled with the utmost care.

How Is Counseling Paid For?

Here again, the answer to this is going to vary by region. Licensed counselors may be able to get insurance reimbursement, usually for a limited period of time. Counselors in private practice as well as agencies can otherwise charge a fee for the service, including a sliding scale. Organizations can get grants and donations with which to set up programs if it's not feasible within existing budgets. It is hoped that eventually Medicare will routinely pay for counseling for PWESD.

There are many settings that could appropriately offer this service. These include dementia care agencies, diagnostic and research centers, mental health centers, area agencies on aging, and universities. Costs include publicity, staff time for intakes and counseling, and printed materials given to PWESD and their families.

The costs of replicating this program depend also upon the level of training needed. More experienced counselors will, of course, need less training. And, new programs have more start-up costs all around than those that become established.

Funding has unfortunately become scarcer for many important social services. And yet, Alzheimer's professionals and advocates continue to have success with policy efforts. The intent here is to offer a clear, well-grounded, and substantial model that can become part of the service schema, modifiable to fit wherever you are.

Working with Other Agencies

The role of other agencies has been touched on earlier but bears repeating. You want to raise awareness within your region of early-stage issues and the counseling being offered. Local professionals can provide referrals and may be called upon to coordinate complex cases with you. They might offer more to families or otherwise have services that go beyond what you are set up to do. And, they are critical for implementing follow-up plans, especially when counseling is time limited.

On the other hand, there is great variability in what's available in different regions, and how qualified these agencies are to effectively help with this population. Continuing education and training can be offered to adult protective services, home care, care management, mental health, and other practitioners. They may be particularly called upon for help with PWESD who live alone, have concurrent physical or mental health conditions, or are in transition to residential care placement.

Counseling in Residential Care Settings

Counseling can be very beneficial in assisted living, nursing homes, and other residential care settings. Some people move in because they have dementia, but others develop it afterward. Not all facilities have dementia units, and PWESD who are otherwise healthy may inappropriately wind up on skilled care units. Even those with dementia units are typically for people who are moderately to severely impaired. People in the early stage, then, live amongst the general population—and this gap can pose some challenges.

This author's early-stage support group model was successfully adapted for residents with memory loss in assisted living.[1] Many issues of the framework were found to be relevant, including identity, independence, and spirituality. Other topics that can be addressed with either group or individual support include the following:

- How moving happened and how the person feels about it

- Pros and cons of living in residential care

- The sense of isolation and being ostracized by others in the facility

- The mystery of and fears about the dementia unit

- What help is available from staff in the building

Providing counseling in residential care facilities may entail additional components, depending upon your time and interests. Multidisciplinary staff from the ground to the top can benefit from training to improve their interactions with PWESD. Education for residents without dementia breaks down barriers of stigma. Support for families, who are often in fear and denial about impairment, makes disclosure and transition between units less difficult. Overall, refuting stereotypes, reframing perceptions, and teaching skills in these settings are some of the challenging but necessary shifts that would make the mental health of PWESD in their care more of a priority. The outcome vitally enhances quality of life as well as the competence of these residential communities.

CHAPTER 13

Pilot Project Evaluation

Project Background

This section tethers all of the tale's previous chapters to the pilot project that initiated it. Funding came from the U.S. Administration on Aging's Alzheimer's Disease Innovation Program to the Georgia Division of Aging Services. As part of the larger grant, the Georgia Chapter of the Alzheimer's Association contracted with Robyn Yale, LCSW, to develop a counseling program, and provide consultation on the clinical and administrative aspects of implementing it. The book's Prologue details more about the project partners and this collaboration. Presented here are sections of the evaluation report by the Georgia Health Policy Center (where indicated), followed by feedback from this author's personal communications with the counselors.

Overview

The counseling model and protocol described in this book were formalized from the start of the two-year project. A daylong training session was then provided to the counselors, the evaluators, and other staff of the Alzheimer's Associations and Area Agencies on Aging in Atlanta and Augusta, Georgia. Following this, screening and selection of appropriate counseling participants were conducted for several months using the tools and procedures explained in Chapter 10.

Counseling began with participants completing a survey that identified their concerns and structured their goals. The survey contained the Framework for Coping with Early Dementia (described in Chapter 2), with its three primary areas of Emotional Adjustment, Practical Coping Strategies, and Lifestyle Issues. Counseling was then provided in eight weekly sessions of 55 minutes each to work on the issues that emerged. Time and funding constraints did not allow families to formally participate in the counseling, but counselees had the option of inviting them in toward the ends of their sessions to discuss certain areas or assignments.

Surveys were readministered in follow-up interviews within two weeks of each participant's last counseling session. Evaluators also asked open-ended questions. The aim was to determine how helpful the participants found counseling to be.

Three counselors administered the counseling. Clinical supervision was provided by this author. At the end of the project, the counselors were also interviewed by the evaluators to get their perspective on the experience.

Counselors and Counselees

Of the seventeen counseling participants discussed, eight were men and nine were women. They ranged in age from early 50s to 80s. The majority were Caucasian, two were African-American, and one was Hispanic. Over half lived in rural areas. As mentioned, they were determined to be willing and able to discuss their diagnosis of AD or other dementia through the screening process before beginning counseling.

All three counselors were female and were either master's-level trained in clinical counseling or a licensed clinical social worker. Each had substantial experience (from 20 to 38 years) providing counseling services. Two of the three also had at least 18 years of experience working specifically with persons with dementia, while one had more limited experience.

The Pre- and Postsurvey Tools

The pre- and postsurveys used in the pilot project were slightly modified from the forms you read about in Chapter 5 (setting clinical counseling goals) and Chapter 11 (evaluating counseling and progress toward goals). They were initially inspired by a discussion with early-stage expert and researcher Linda Clare, with further consultation from early-stage researcher Scott Roberts.

Clare had studied the clinical efficacy of cognitive rehabilitation in early-stage AD.[1] The levels of performance and satisfaction on personalized goals were rated after an eight-week intervention. Clare adapted the Canadian Occupational

Performance Measure (COPM) developed by Law et al.[2] for use in her randomized clinical trial. Categories of concerns included self-care, productivity, and leisure.

This approach of formulating individualized goals to develop treatment and evaluation plans fit nicely with the structure of the coping framework in this project. Counseling and evaluation staff took the templates designed here and added on rating scales with multiple response categories for their use. That is, the evaluators asked questions to understand if the intervention was very helpful, somewhat helpful, or not helpful in addressing the identified areas of concern. The participants could also give open-ended responses to these items and to other questions about their overall experience with the intervention.

Results from the Formal Evaluation

The following sections (through footnote #3) are excerpted with permission from the project report.

A. Recipients of Counseling Services: Persons with Early-Stage Alzheimer's Disease or Other Dementia

The participants felt very positive about the counseling program, and the success of addressing their concerns. All were very satisfied with the counseling they received and said that they would recommend the program to others. The evaluators identified several areas within the three primary areas of the Framework for Coping with Early Dementia that the participants indicated were "very helpful":

Emotional Adjustment: *Expressing Feelings*

The participants explained that the opportunity to talk about their diagnosis, disease, and the multitude of emotions that they were going through at this time was highly valuable. In addition, the importance of a nonjudgmental atmosphere, provided by a counselor with subject matter expertise, was essential in creating a safe environment for sharing their feelings. One participant stated, *"This program has been a lifeline for me, really. I don't know what I would have done without it. I think I can make it now."*

Practical Coping Strategies: *Memory Aids*

Learning skills to assist in dealing with day-to-day challenges of memory loss was a particularly important part of the counseling. Many participants discussed learning new systems for managing their day or keeping track of their thoughts, and then utilizing these strategies with immediate success or improvement. A participant commented: *"[The program] helped me become more adventurous in my kitchen. Now I make lists and that is really helpful."* Another explained to his counselor that he could not keep track of the holidays and remember to get cards for his wife, which led to a tremendous feeling of inadequacy as a husband. The counselor [suggested] purchasing a calendar with pockets for each month in which to place holiday cards. This aid enabled the man to give cards to his wife throughout the year.

Practical Coping Strategies: *Cognitive Exercise*

Addressing concerns over increasing memory loss, participants found cognitive exercises to be useful tools. Some of the exercises they mentioned trying included puzzles, word games, trivia games, and video games. One said that these activities are *"good at keeping me sharp and quick."* Several participants showed the evaluators the puzzles and games, and talked about the benefit of keeping their minds "active."

Lifestyle Issues: *Family Relationships*

Many of the participants discussed the difficulties they had in communicating with family members about their disease or the changes that may be necessary in the near future. Many expressed hesitance to share their concerns/fears with family members who had their "own stuff" to deal with, and the individual did not want to add to their burden. Spouses did not want to worry each other; and parents did not want to share their fears with their children, because they felt that their role was to protect their children, not to worry them. There were also several accounts of individuals trying to share their diagnosis with family members; however, when they did so, family members seemed unable to hear it. Some recounted receiving responses such as "Oh Mom, you're okay" or "That's just what happens when you age." Counseling recipients shared with the evaluators their belief that family members are often in denial and may need counseling services of their own. Counseling provided the participants the opportunity to talk about the dynamics that shape familial relationships. Several stated they may not have been resolved, but they found it helpful to talk with the counselor about these issues.

Lifestyle Issues: *Service Utilization*

Bringing an awareness of the resources that are available to persons with early-stage dementia was discussed as very helpful to many participants. Consumption of recommended reading, attending educational programs, and utilization of support groups, senior centers, and social groups were seen as highly valuable. One participant described his experience in an art class where he drew a picture that presented his view of the effects of dementia on his body, which he explained was a powerful experience for both himself and other people in the class.

Logistical Factors

Two logistical factors were raised by participants as important to the success of the program. First was the quality of the counselors, [who were seen as] well-informed, knowledgeable, easy to talk to, and a safe place to share feelings. Secondly, most participants had the counseling sessions in their homes, which they reflected made the program accessible to them and made them feel supported. One participant stated: *"In-home was the best. In your home, you are more secure and able to face facts."* For people with dementia, the home environment seems to support recall and memory, along with being a place of emotional familiarity and security. This is not to say that if the program were held outside the home, none would be able to participate; however, the home location was preferable for many of the individuals interviewed.

The following were responses to open-ended questions:

Which part of the counseling was most helpful to you?

"It helped me to still be a husband to my wife."

"[The counselor] helped me go over things that I have never thought of, things about cleaning, and making a schedule and other things around the house. . . . I enjoyed it every time she came over."

"Getting information about dementia, I learned a lot about the disease that I did not learn from the neurologist."

"The counselor was my guardian angel."

Which part of the counseling was least helpful to you?

"I enjoyed every minute of it."

"Maybe we could have had more sessions."

What could be added or changed in the counseling program to make it better?

"It would depend on the person you're talking to. Other people may need additional sessions in order to loosen up."

"It couldn't have helped me anymore."

"I would like to talk to a peer to learn about their experience."

"The quality of the counselor is very important. Mine was very good. I recommend a mature counselor so that they can bring the knowledge of age with them."

B. Clinical Counseling Providers

Each counselor stated that she felt the service addressed an often unmet need—that is, a structured way of providing support and information to individuals in the early stages of Alzheimer's disease or other dementias.

Each counselor reported a positive experience, both from a career and a personal perspective. One said it was an *"honor"* to be invited into people's homes and lives at a time of such transition for them. Another said, *"It was a tremendously positive experience, and I was glad to be a part of it."*

When asked if there were particular areas that seemed to be most beneficial to participants, counselors cited both the overall structure of the counseling protocol (recognizing the dimensions of coping) and specific resources, such as the Critical Pathways book, which documents finances, living wills, and plans for the future. The flexible protocol allowed the counselors to focus on the areas most beneficial to each particular client; this was especially important since they were working within a short time frame.

Each counselor mentioned the unique combination of skills necessary to provide high-quality services to persons with early dementia. *"It is important to have someone providing the Clinical Counseling Program who has a dementia background as well as counseling skills. Matching the participant and the counselor for the most effective combination is important."*

Effective screening of potential participants is also important. *"For this counseling to be most effective, the client needs to be very early-stage, have some acceptance of what is going on, and not have unmet mental health needs."*

Although all the counselors described overwhelmingly positive experiences, there were suggestions of ways to strengthen the protocol and the program in the future.

- There was a general feeling of the importance/necessity of involving caretakers and family members in some structured way during the counseling process. Although the uniqueness of this program is the focus on the individual, family members/caretakers are integral parts of their lives and there should be appropriate roles for them in the counseling sessions.

- The suggestion was also made that the 55-minute time limit for each session should be amended to provide for longer therapy. In addition, counselors felt that the number of sessions provided should be based on need, rather than a set number.

- One counselor stated that she realized with budget constraints and personnel limitations, sessions could not be unlimited; and the suggestion was made that after the conclusion of the counseling program structured follow-up be provided to the individuals; for example, a call in the month following the final counseling session, and depending on need, additional follow-ups every two to three months.

C. Research Lessons Learned

In the first year of the evaluation, the interviews were conducted either by phone, video conferencing, or in person. At the end of the first round of interviews, the evaluators determined that when conducting an interview in person, they are more likely to be able to discern if an individual becomes confused or is unable to follow the questions. In the second year, all interviews were conducted in person.

This type of evaluation requires researchers/evaluators to understand some of the issues that surround gathering information from individuals with memory loss. For example, recall is often difficult. Being in a familiar setting (such as a home setting) can sometimes help. Other strategies include using pictures to stimulate memory. In this study, it would have been helpful to have pictures of the counselors to show individuals as they were being interviewed about the clinical counseling sessions. Visual cues may be especially important for people with memory loss who are involved in multiple support programs.

Working with universities' internal review boards (IRBs) can be time consuming when gaining approval for any projects involving people with memory loss. They are considered a vulnerable population and special precautions are taken to insure their rights are protected during the evaluation process. Gaining consent from individuals with memory loss should be ongoing and evaluators should not assume that because consent was given at the beginning of the process, the individual remembers giving that consent about involvement in the evaluation. The conversations about the purpose of the interview should happen repeatedly.

D. Conclusion

The clinical counseling program appears to have been successful in addressing many of the areas of concern that were identified by the participants interviewed. Numerous participants remarked on the difficulty of handling the diagnosis of early-stage AD and the feeling of leaving the doctor's office with little information on the disease or what to do next. The number of participants self-identifying as concerned about areas relating to emotional adjustment, and interested in the coping strategies and lifestyle issues, indicates the importance of the clinical counseling program in bridging the gap after diagnosis. Although they did not often feel that their physicians provided them with much information about the implications of their diagnosis, participants still identified physicians as being important sources of information; consequently, partnering with diagnosing physicians could lead to increased outreach for the program in the future.

The quality and experience of counselors was key in the positive experiences of the participants, and will determine the success of this protocol in the future. With appropriately trained and experienced counselors, it is apparent that this clinical counseling protocol can provide much needed support and guidance during difficult transition points in people's lives. A diagnosis of Alzheimer's disease carries serious and complicated issues surrounding emotional adjustment and coping, as well as practical issues such as financial planning and decisions around whether/how to inform employers, family members, etc. To be effective in the role of counseling individuals with early-stage Alzheimer's disease, counselors need to understand the gravity and possible implications of these emotions and decisions, and be able to refer them to experts (law, tax attorneys for example) when necessary.[3]

Results from Consultation with Project Staff

The following sections (through footnote #4) are based on communications between this author and the project's three counselors in consultation sessions.

Types of Cases

Generally speaking, the types of counseling cases demonstrated that while the focus might be on one area of the Framework for Coping with Early Dementia, the others were also integral to the effort. Referring back to the goal sheets in Chapter 5, we can look at a few examples of this. One gentleman who was isolated due to retiring found new meaning and purpose (Emotional) in volunteering (Lifestyle) to provide peer phone support to other early-stage individuals (Practical). At the same time, he was connected to several local early-stage recreational programs (Lifestyle). And, a woman who was depressed upon learning her diagnosis found it helpful to process her feelings (Emotional). She was also referred for an antidepressant to a mental health provider (Lifestyle), attended an early-stage support group (Lifestyle), started singing and exercise activities (Practical); and her family was brought into the counseling for education and support (Lifestyle).

A. Counseling Recipients

When asked for feedback from the counseling participants, the counselors provided the following quotes. It was clear that some of the PWESD had been struggling with tremendous fear:

"You literally saved my life. I had pills in my house and had many thoughts of taking them because I was so afraid of what would happen next in my life."

"I have been most afraid of having to leave my home and becoming a vegetable in a nursing home. You've shown me that I can stay at home and when the time is right have help to stay here even longer. I never knew that even with something this devastating I can still go on. Thank you."

"I have several degrees, have managed many programs and large groups of people, but nothing has prepared me for this (Alzheimer's disease). I now have a greater understanding of why I was so afraid and of the path this disease will take. I now have new strategies to use when my emotions get the best of me."

"You get your diagnosis and a prescription, and the doctor says to come back in six months. So you're left thinking, 'Now what?' It's a very scary feeling. The counseling has been tremendously helpful, informative, and reassuring to me, and I hope it will become available to more people in my situation."

Other PWESD talked about the palpable sense of loss and aloneness they'd been experiencing:

"I think this counseling is very important, because you need someone to talk to when you get this diagnosis—but very few people really understand it or what it's like to go through it."

"The counseling has made me feel less alone, and more hopeful."

"My psychiatrist is very impressed with my progress during the past few months and has even cut my medication down. I am not as depressed as I was in April."

And several PWESD incorporated comments about their families into the way counseling helped them understand their situations and feel better about themselves:

"My greatest loss was feeling that I could no longer contribute to my family. You showed me how to celebrate even small accomplishments by writing them on a calendar and seeing all I really do in a week. Thank you for making me feel like a man again."

"My family has never accepted my memory issues. You have helped me and them to see this situation in a new way. I think we will be alright now."

"Thank you for letting me talk about my feelings and fears in my own way. My family loves me but often finish my sentences and don't really listen to me. You truly understand and offered great new ways to think about myself and my future."

One family member was also quoted at the end of the project:

"Since my mom lives alone, I am so grateful there is a program to help her realize she will need to come live in my home at some point. After you began working with her, she seems more willing to look at her future with us."

B. Counseling Providers

When the counselors were asked for feedback, they talked about how the experience touched them:

"Counseling one of our participants was one of the most profoundly moving experiences of my professional life; I felt privileged to witness her capacity for accepting her Alzheimer's and continuing to live her life with joy. To just be with her while she panicked, surrendered, and then found her way back . . . "

"It was very rewarding to see a physical change in several PWESD as they found new self-worth, meaning and hope in their lives. Individuals

changed in presentation, affect, posture and grooming; one began to smile more, and one family member said her mother cried less. Several who always wanted to stay in accompanied spouses to public activities (church, shopping) more."

"This gave me a different perspective with which to handle calls."

"I found this fascinating, and I hope the program continues as a cutting-edge approach."

"The program has made a real difference in the lives of the people I have counseled. It's my sincere hope that this counseling protocol will be learned and adopted nationwide."

C. Lessons Learned

Project staff also discussed issues that came up for them in doing the counseling:

- The large and rural geographic region was a concern for participants who would have to drive great distances to come to an office. The counselors chose to do home visits, which increased the time needed to provide the service.

- Time was also required that had not been completely anticipated for the length of the screening and intake process, extra calls outside of counseling sessions, and contact with families.

- The eight-week pilot period was seen as too short by the counselors. It was difficult to disengage at that point and follow-up needed to be built in.

- Counselors saw that having dementia happens on top of other crises and things going on in people's lives. PWESD's challenges are complex and multifaceted (especially those living alone), and often fall into the realm of care management. Examples include medical care/medications, financial information due to loss of income and insurance, family/marital issues, safety, relocation, transportation, and protective services. There are many unmet needs and few resources.

- It was understood that the project didn't have funding to incorporate counseling for families. But the realization came that there were also few counselors to refer to in the community who were truly well trained in early dementia.[4]

Conclusion

This was an initial effort to evaluate the new counseling program. The pilot project's results speak to the model being feasible, therapeutic, and warranting further study. The acceptance of new interventions is best bolstered by quantitative research, with its challenging design and methodological parameters. Chapter 5 and

Chapter 11 contain sections that refer further to this. It is hoped that investigators with the requisite experience and skills will be interested in attempting to correlate counseling goals with appropriate outcome measures. This will take the assessment of improved coping in the three areas of the framework to the next level.

The model is now systematized, and the book developed so that others can replicate it. At the same time, it's adaptable to various settings and formats depending upon how it can best be implemented in any particular region. Whether dementia care agencies provide counseling themselves or partner with other practitioners to offer it, training needs to happen and the service expanded. This will also facilitate the opportunity for additional research in the future.

Having reflected on the pilot project, we arrive next at the "denouement"—which the dictionary defines as the final revelation of the plot of a tale.

CHAPTER 14

Denouement

Fitting It All Together

When you put your hand into a flowing stream,
you touch the last that has gone before
and the first of what is still to come

—Leonardo da Vinci

The Arc of a Story

Tales are most satisfying when the pieces of the puzzle they present fit together at the end. We began with the metaphors of revolution and evolution as the basis of powerful transformation on multiple levels. These dynamic processes allow us to battle AD with new understandings and approaches, across the fields of multiple disciplines. Counseling builds an individualized ally into this increasingly sophisticated arsenal.

The arc of an interesting story consists of threads that are woven through it and pulled out the other side. Its characters are presented with choices as they confront calamity. We hope that in the end they find the wisdom and strength to resolve their conflicts, but sometimes we are parted without ever knowing what becomes of them.

In this tale, people go through the arc of the Framework for Coping with Early Dementia, with its interconnected emotional, practical, and lifestyle doorways. It's been constructed with the solid materials of well-credentialed counselors and a process by which only those who can handle this particular journey are invited to enter. Together, we establish a grounding relationship, explore the numerous challenges, and carve a path through the labyrinth of their multilayered issues. It takes all of our skills—and all of theirs.

It's nice when tales have happy endings. But many times they don't. In fiction, fantasy, fairy tales, fables, and in actual fact: Life is perilous. It's full of unforeseeable heartache and drama, change and trauma. But it's also full of wonder, beauty, joy, and amazing feats of triumph over adversity.

As counselors, we really can't walk in the moccasins of the person with dementia. We can look at the slice of life occurring right now and we can peer around the possible corners of the future. We can listen and reflect, raise awareness and make suggestions, put plans and linkages in place that will all hopefully help them manage. They will still have the disease, but they will also still have their personhood. We recognize it because we each have our struggles. We respond because we all need to feel valued in spite of them.

So, we are back where we started, having come full circle. I've aimed for a sense of completion, as well as a readiness to begin anew. As T. S. Eliot wrote:

> We shall not cease from exploration
>
> And the end of all our exploring
>
> Will be to arrive where we started
>
> And know the place for the first time.[1]

The Arc of Revolution

Tales are most intriguing when they tell of a quest. And, when we witness others becoming more fully themselves in the face of seemingly insurmountable odds. The words of the writer Anne Lamott fit well here, when she says: *Hope is a revolutionary patience.*[2]

Revolution can be heralded by a battle cry across the land—forceful and loud. Or it can have a quiet, internal power like that of the martial arts warrior. It does take a certain boldness for people with dementia to speak their truth, to believe in their abilities, and to advocate for themselves. They must fight to defy conventional norms and stereotypes while also victoriously capturing their own inner reserves. They must persevere with faith and forbearance.

The counselor who joins forces with PWESD—catalyzing and strategizing—also engages in a revolutionary act. It takes tremendous wholeheartedness and fortitude just to be present. Serving as a refuge for those displaced by the avalanche of a dementia diagnosis, we shelter their fears and hopes, disappointments and dreams at a time of great vulnerability. We must match their authenticity and determination with our own dedication. We nurture their resilience, while also attempting to alter the attitudes, beliefs, and systems around us. Together, we spark progressive social change. It might even be powerful enough to shift the orbits of dementia care, research, science, and policy more into alignment with what's needed—and with one another.

The Arc of Evolution

Tales are most motivating when they show us a way forward. When PWESD grow in self-esteem; when they and their families can make better connections between the parts of their lives and more skillfully address them; when counselors and counselees are raising the consciousness of those in the field and the larger society; when organizational and national plans are incorporating the input of PWESD into their missions and standards of care, we are collectively improving quality of life. Metamorphosis on these multiple levels may be slow. But that is truly evolution in action.

All forms of life must continually adapt if they are to survive. At times of change and crisis, we all reexamine our priorities. We rely on our inner resources as well as the caring of others to help us recalibrate and remain engaged in life.

At the axis of a dementia diagnosis, there is much that can't be controlled. But one can take command of the interpretation and reaction to having the condition. Right now, there is no possibility of an immediate cure, so tools to cope with it are essential. This is true of the ubiquitous challenges we all face. We have to determine which things we can do something about, and which we must come to terms with and accept.

As a counselor, you will also evolve when you practice this intervention. The effort required to establish the new service takes a huge commitment. It gives back immeasurable reward. Navigating in a new clinical direction sharpens our skills, and deepens us.

The Arc of Transformation

Tales are most compelling when transformation occurs. Dementia is life changing, but so is what happens in response to it. There are different ways of drawing lessons from stories. If the main characters have moved us, they resonate and stay with us. The morals of this narrative are that PWESD don't have to be conquered by misfortune. They can transcend it. And that their situations, while each unique, all reflect to us our common humanity.

In reading this book, you must have been on a quest as well. I hope you've learned a bit about helping PWESD maximize their potential and find meaning even in the face of disease progression. Perhaps you've also reflected upon the universal demand that we adjust to whatever happens in our lives. We all seek avenues for happiness and fulfillment even when roadblocks appear during times of great transition.

In the sacred space of the counseling relationship, both counselor and counselee are enriched and transformed. Each is meant to give and to receive. Digging deep into emotional trenches is intense work. It simultaneously softens and toughens us. We become more open, less intimidated, and quite sure of the brute force of our capabilities.

I trust that following this tale has altered your outlook and intentions. Even if you won't be the one to do counseling, maybe you'll be inspired to collaborate with others around you to make it happen. May this book fortify you in the task of more effectively assisting PWESD, and on your own personal journey. Please take a page from my book, and step forward with confidence. I wish you well.

And now, the tale's Epilogue.

Epilogue

If there is no wind, row.

—Latin proverb

Before I committed to writing this book, a good friend of mine (whom I'll call Linda) was strongly encouraging me to do it. She then offered a lot of support as I undertook the project. I've known her for many years, and it so happens that she's been experiencing memory loss for some time. As I was finishing the book, she took to heart my encouragement to get this checked out, and finally went to the doctor. He was at a major HMO in the San Francisco Bay Area, which is a relatively sophisticated and service-rich region in terms of dementia care.

Linda was sent to a neurologist who told her that she had MCI. He patted her on the head, saying it was a good thing that impairment hadn't progressed much since it began. He discouraged treatment with medication, saying that what's available doesn't work. He sent her home without any literature, referrals to appropriate agencies, suggestions for optimizing functioning or cognitive health, or plans for follow-up evaluation.

When she relayed this to me, I called several colleagues to talk it over. A social worker in the local diagnostic center felt that the MCI diagnosis is often used to spare people's feelings, rather than enabling them to confront having dementia. She also commented that more patients in her setting are asking tough questions about incapacity and related matters in a way they weren't five or ten years ago. Though she herself has been working with dementia caregivers for many years, she needs guidance and support to honestly answer these queries from PWESD.

The staff at the regional Alzheimer's Association have heard other stories like Linda's about this particular HMO, and offered ideas and referrals. We theorized that routinely not prescribing medications saves the provider money. We discussed how the new diagnostic guidelines can keep doctors from making certain recommendations that they would have for a diagnosis of early dementia when instead the label is MCI. It's also clear that the shift in emphasis from early-stage AD to MCI expands the pool of people that is available to researchers. Research is certainly critical. But that is a tale for another time.

And Linda? For the moment she seems to be doing what many do now when told that they have MCI, which is avoiding identifying with dementia. I don't push her on it. However, I'm seeking the name of a good specialist within her HMO as she'd like to get a second opinion about trying the medication.

I found it ironic that a friend of mine had this experience, and responded as she did, while I was writing this tome. But I shouldn't be surprised. I'm sure that everyone who is reading this knows of someone in a similar situation. It strengthens my resolve to create better alternatives—for doctors, for other care providers, and for people who are going through it.

The late African-American tennis champion and humanitarian Arthur Ashe had this to say about being a trailblazer. It seems like a good ending to the story of counselors and PWESD: *Start where you are. Use what you have. Do what you can.*

And finally, a few words of thanks: First, this book wouldn't have been possible without the respectful trust placed in me by the Georgia Chapter of the Alzheimer's Association, and the funding they provided. Secondly, their project staff (named in the Prologue) made a critical footprint on a new path for others to follow. Third, their (and all of my previous) counselees have been sage mentors whose courage imparts to us an important legacy.

Fourth, I greatly appreciate this book's publisher, Health Professions Press, for their interest in my new work, for providing their expert assistance in bringing my vision forward, and for expediting its production for my training workshops.

Next, I extend deep bows of gratitude to my husband, David, for his wisdom, equanimity, and steady support while this new work of mine was being born. And, I'm thrilled that his beautiful photo graces the book's cover!

Lastly, I thank you, the reader—for giving the tale a listen, and for all you may already be doing on the front lines every single day.

REFERENCES

Chapter 1. Introduction: Looking Back and Forward

1. Yale, R. (1995). *Support Groups for Individuals with Early-Stage Alzheimer's Disease: Planning, Implementation, and Evaluation.* Baltimore, MD: Health Professions Press.

2. Alzheimer's Disease International. (1991 & 2002). *Charter of Principles.* London. Retrieved from www.alz.co.uk/charter-of-principals

3. Reed, P. & Bluethmann, S. (2008). *Voices of Alzheimer's' Disease: A Summary Report on the Nationwide Town Hall Meetings for People with Early-Stage Dementia.* Chicago, IL: Alzheimer's Association.

4. National Institutes of Health, National Institute on Aging, Alzheimer's Disease Education and Referral Center. *Diagnostic Guidelines for Alzheimer's Disease: Frequently Asked Questions for Clinicians.* Retrieved from http://www.nia.nih.gov/alzheimers/diagnostic-guidelines-alzheimers-disease-frequently-asked-questions-clinicians

5. Rettner, R. (2012, February 7). New Alzheimer's criteria would change diagnosis for millions. *Live Science News.* Retrieved from http://news.yahoo.com/alzheimers-criteria-change-diagnosis-millions-214203482.html

6. Kolata, G. (2010, July 13). Rules seek to expand diagnosis of Alzheimer's. *The New York Times.* Retrieved from http://www.nytimes.com/2010/07/14/health/policy/14alzheimer.html

Chapter 3. Identifying the Special Issues and Challenges Facing People with Early-Stage Dementia

1. Livni, M. (2010). *The Japanese Therapists: Another Alzheimer's Autobiography.* Saxonwold, SA: Michael Livni.

2. Yale, R. (1995). *Support Groups for Individuals with Early-Stage Alzheimer's Disease: Planning, Implementation, and Evaluation.* Baltimore, MD: Health Professions Press.

Chapter 4. The Counseling Approach and Relationship

1. Yale, R. (1995). *Support Groups for Individuals with Early-Stage Alzheimer's Disease: Planning, Implementation, and Evaluation.* Baltimore, MD: Health Professions Press.

2. Yalom, I. (2002). *The Gift of Therapy.* New York, NY: Harper Collins.

3. Seligman, M. (2011). *Flourish: A Visionary New Understanding of Happiness and Well-Being.* New York, NY: Free Press.

4. Kornfield, J. (2008). *The Wise Heart*. New York, NY: Bantam Books.

5. Association for Humanistic Psychology. *Our New Vision*. Retrieved from www.ahpweb.org

6. Rogers, C.R. (1951). *Client-Centered Therapy*. Boston, MA: Houghton Mifflin.

7. Kitwood, T. (1997). *Dementia Reconsidered: The Person Comes First*. Buckingham: Open University Press.

8. Yale, R. (1989). Support groups for newly-diagnosed Alzheimer's clients. *Clinical Gerontologist*, 8(3), 86–89.

9. Yalom, I. (1995). *The Theory and Practice of Group Psychotherapy* (Fourth Edition). New York, NY: Basic Books.

10. Yale, R. (1995). *Support Groups for Individuals with Early-Stage Alzheimer's Disease: Planning, Implementation, and Evaluation*. Baltimore, MD: Health Professions Press.

11. Cohen, G. (1988). One psychiatrist's view. In L. Jarvik & C. Winograd (Eds.) *Treatments for the Alzheimer's Patient: The Long Haul*. New York, NY: Springer, 96–104.

12. Sabat, S. (2001). *The Experience of Alzheimer's Disease: Life Through A Tangled Veil*. Malden, MA: Blackwell Publishers.

13. Snyder, L. (2009). *Speaking Our Minds—What It's Like to Have Alzheimer's* (Revised Edition). Baltimore, MD: Health Professions Press.

14. Yale, R. & Kaplan, D. (2006). Memory loss support groups for residents of assisted living: Enhancing quality of care and quality of life. *Alzheimer's Care Quarterly*, 7(4), 226–242.

15. Livni, M. (2010). *The Japanese Therapists: Another Alzheimer's Autobiography*. Saxonwold, SA: Michael Livni.

16. Murray Alzheimer's Research & Education Program. (2008). *By Us For Us Guides*. Ontario: University of Waterloo. Retrieved from http://www.marep.uwaterloo.ca/products/bufu.html

17. Morhardt, D. (2004). Top 10 ideas for enhancing quality of life by diagnosed individuals and families living with Alzheimer's and related dementias. *Alzheimer's Care Quarterly*, 5(2), 103–107.

18. South West Dementia Partnerships. (2011). *Making Involvement Count: Involving People Living with Dementia Resource Pack*. Bristol, UK: Dementia Partnerships South West.

19. McKillop, J. & Wilkinson, H. (2004). Make it easy on yourself: Advice to researchers from someone with dementia on being interviewed. *Dementia*, 3(2), 117–125.

20. Yale, R. (1995). *Support Groups for Individuals with Early-Stage Alzheimer's Disease: Planning, Implementation, and Evaluation*. Baltimore, MD: Health Professions Press.

21. Cheston, R., Jones, K., & Gilliard, J. (2003). Group psychotherapy and people with dementia. *Aging & Mental Health*, 7(6), 452–461.

22. Clare, L. (2002). We'll fight it as long as we can: Coping with the onset of Alzheimer's disease. *Aging & Mental Health,* 6(2), 139–148.

23. Keady, J. & Nolan, M. (1995). IMMEL2: Working to augment coping responses in early dementia. *British Journal of Nursing,* 4(7), 377–380.

24. Holst, G. & Hallberg, I. (2003). Exploring the meaning of everyday life for those suffering from dementia. *American Journal of Alzheimers' Disease and Other Dementias,* 18(6), 359–365.

25. Roberts, J.S. & Silverio, E. (2009). Evaluation of an education and support program for early-stage Alzheimer's disease. *Journal of Applied Gerontology,* 28(4), 419–435.

26. Zarit, S., Femia, E., Watson, J., Rice-Oeschger, L., & Kakos, B. (2004). Memory club: A group intervention for people with early-stage dementia and their care partners. *The Gerontologist,* 44(2), 262–269.

27. Clare, L., Linden, D., Woods, R., Whitaker, R., Evans, S., Parkinson, C., van Paasschen, J., Nelis, S., Hoare, Z., Yuen, K., & Rugg, M. (2010). Goal-oriented cognitive rehabilitation for people with early-stage Alzheimer disease: A single-blind randomized controlled trial of clinical efficacy. *American Journal of Geriatric Psychiatry,* 18(10), 928–939.

28. Bird, M., Caldwell, T., Maller, J., & Korten, A. (2005). *Alzheimer's Australia Early-Stage Dementia Support & Respite Project: Final Evaluation Report.* Commonwealth of Australia.

29. Roberts, J.S. & Silverio, E. (2009). Evaluation of an education and support program for early-stage Alzheimer's disease. *Journal of Applied Gerontology,* 28(4), 419–435.

30. Woods, B. (2010). Non-pharmacological therapies. *Global Perspective—Newsletter of Alzheimer's Disease International,* 20(5), p. 11.

31. Moniz-Cook, E., Vernooij-Dassen, M., Woods, B., Orrell, M., & Interdem Network. (2011). Psychosocial interventions in dementia care research: The Interdem manifesto. *Aging & Mental Health,* 15(3), 283–290.

32. Bunn, F., Goodman, C., Sworn, K., Rait, G., Brayne, C., Robinson, L., McNeilly, E., & Iliffe, S. (2012). Psychosocial factors that shape patient and carer experiences of dementia diagnosis and treatment: A systematic review of qualitative studies. *Public Library of Science—Medicine,* 9(10), doi: 10.1371/journal.pmed1001331

33. Prince, M., Bryce, R., & Ferri, C. (2011). *World Alzheimer Report 2011: The Benefits of Early Diagnosis and Intervention.* London: Alzheimer's Disease International.

34. Batsch, N. & Mittelman, M. (2012). *World Alzheimer Report 2012: Overcoming the Stigma of Dementia.* London: Alzheimer's Disease International.

35. U.S. Department of Health & Human Services. (2012). *National Plan to Address Alzheimer's Disease.* Retrieved from aspe.hhs.gov/daltcp/napa/natlplan.shtml

36. Cole, D. (2012). Is psychotherapy getting better? *Psychotherapy Networker,* 36(2), p. 24.

37. Yalom, I. (2002). *The Gift of Therapy.* New York, NY: Harper Collins.

38. Geda, Y. (2010). Mayo Clinic study finds apathy and depression predict progression from mild cognitive impairment to dementia. *Mayo Clinic News*. Retrieved from http://www.mayoclinic.org/news2010-rst/5857.html

39. Yalom, I. (1995). *The Theory and Practice of Group Psychotherapy* (Fourth Edition). New York, NY: Basic Books.

40. Yale, R. (1995). *Support Groups for Individuals with Early-Stage Alzheimer's Disease: Planning, Implementation, and Evaluation*. Baltimore, MD: Health Professions Press.

Chapter 6. Addressing the Special Issues and Challenges Facing People with Early-Stage Dementia

1. Yale, R. (1995). *Support Groups for Individuals with Early-Stage Alzheimer's Disease: Planning, Implementation, and Evaluation*. Baltimore, MD: Health Professions Press.

2. Bordisso, L. (2012). Here and now. *Perspectives—A Newsletter for Individuals with Alzheimer's or a Related Disorder*, 17(2), p. 1.

3. Snyder, L. (2012). Brainstorming: Managing frustration. *Perspectives—A Newsletter for Individuals with Alzheimer's or a Related Disorder*, 17(3), p. 3.

4. Warner, M. & Warner, E. (2000). *The Complete Guide to Alzheimer's-Proofing Your Home* (Revised Edition). West Lafayette, IN: Purdue University Press.

5. Murray Alzheimer's Research and Education Program. (2008). *Enhancing Communication—A By Us For Us Guide*. Ontario: University of Waterloo.

6. Alzheimer's Association. *Maintain Your Brain*. Retrieved November 11, 2012, from http://www.alz.org/we_can_help_brain_health_maintain_your_brain.asp

7. Emerson Lombardo, N. (2012). Alzheimer's disease. In J. Rippe (Ed.), *Encyclopedia of Lifestyle Medicine and Health*. Thousand Oaks, CA: Sage Press, 120–142.

8. Einberger, K. & Sellick, J. (2006). *Strengthen Your Mind: Activities for People with Early Memory Loss*. Baltimore, MD: Health Professions Press.

9. Murray Alzheimer's Research and Education Program. (2008). *Living and Celebrating Life Through Leisure—A By Us For Us Guide*. Ontario: University of Waterloo.

10. Warner, C. (2012). Plan for the future but live in the "now." *Perspectives— A Newsletter for Individuals with Alzheimer's or a Related Disorder*, 17(4), p. 4.

11. Yale, R. & Snyder, L. (2002). The experience of support groups for persons with early-stage Alzheimer's disease and their families. In P. Harris (Ed.), *The Person With Alzheimer's Disease: Pathways to Understanding the Experience*. Baltimore, MD: Johns Hopkins University Press, 228–245.

12. Whitlatch, C., Judge, K., Zarit, S., & Femia, E. (2006). Dyadic intervention for family caregivers and care receivers in early-stage dementia. *The Gerontologist*, 46(5), 688–694.

13. Alzheimer's Association, Northern California Chapter. (2011). *Help and Hope: For Persons Diagnosed with Alzheimer's Disease and Related Disorders*. Retrieved from www.alz.org/norcal/documents/06-2011_earlystage_helpandhopehandbook.pdf

14. Snyder, L. (2010). *Living Your Best with Early-Stage Alzheimer's: An Essential Guide.* North Branch MN: Sunrise River Press.

15. Yale, R. (1995). *Support Groups for Individuals with Early-Stage Alzheimer's Disease: Planning, Implementation, and Evaluation.* Baltimore, MD: Health Professions Press.

16. The Hartford. (2007). *At the Crossroads: Family Conversations about Alzheimer's Disease, Dementia and Driving.* Southington, CT: The Hartford.

Chapter 7. The Role of the Family

1. Alzheimer's Association. (2012). Alzheimer's disease facts and figures. *Alzheimer's & Dementia* 8(2).

2. Family Caregiver Alliance. (2003). *Taking Care of YOU: Self-Care for Family Caregivers (Fact Sheet).* San Francisco, CA: Family Caregiver Alliance.

3. Meier Hamilton, J. (2012). Go for it! Self-care is not selfish. *Care Advantage* (Winter Issue). New York, NY: Alzheimer's Foundation of America.

4. Yale, R. (1995). *Support Groups for Individuals with Early-Stage Alzheimer's Disease: Planning, Implementation, and Evaluation.* Baltimore, MD: Health Professions Press.

5. Snyder, L. (2007). Caring for each other: Facing memory loss together. *Perspectives—A Newsletter for Individuals with Alzheimer's or a Related Disorder*, 12(2), p. 1.

6. Michels, B. (2012, October 29). Alzheimer's broke his silence. *Salon.com.* Retrieved from http://www.salon.com/2012/10/29/alzheimer's_broke_his_silence/

7. McKillop, J. (2010). Does dementia affect family relationships? *Global Perspective— Newsletter of Alzheimer's Disease International*, 20(5), p. 10.

8. Steinberg, C. (2012). Talking with Tyler. *Care Advantage* (Spring Issue). New York, NY: Alzheimer's Foundation of America.

9. Alzheimer Europe. (2012). European working group of people with dementia meets for first time in Vienna. *Alzheimer Europe Newsletter* (October Issue). Retrieved from www.alzheimer-europe.org/Publications/newsletters/2012

Chapter 9. Reaching Out to Find Counseling Participants

1. Jenkins, S. (2011, August 23). Pat Summitt, Tennessee women's basketball coach, diagnosed with Alzheimer's disease. *Washington Post.* Retrieved from www.washingtonpost.com/sports/colleges/pat-summitt-tennessee-womens-basketball-coach-diagnosed-with-alzheimers-disease/2011/08/23/g

2. Alzheimer's Disease International. (2003). *How to Include People with Dementia in the Activities of Alzheimer Associations* (Fact Sheet). London: Alzheimer's Disease International.

3. South West Dementia Partnerships. (2011). *Making Involvement Count: Involving People Living with Dementia Resource Pack.* Bristol, UK: Dementia Partnerships South West.

Chapter 10. Assessing and Enrolling Counseling Participants

1. Yale, R. (1995). *Support Groups for Individuals with Early-Stage Alzheimer's Disease: Planning, Implementation, and Evaluation*. Baltimore, MD: Health Professions Press.

2. Alzheimer's Association. (2011). *Telling the Truth in Diagnosis* (Fact Sheet). Chicago, IL: Alzheimer's Association.

3. Prince, M., Bryce, R., & Ferri, C. (2011). *World Alzheimer Report 2011: The Benefits of Early Diagnosis and Intervention*. London: Alzheimer's Disease International.

4. Folstein, M.F., Folstein, S., & McHugh, P.R. (1975). Mini-Mental State: A practical method for grading the cognitive status of patients for the clinician. *Journal of Psychiatric Research* (12), 189–198.

5. Borson, S., Scanlan, J., Brush, M., Vitallano, P., & Dokmak, A. (2000). The Mini-Cog: A cognitive "vital signs" measure for dementia screening in multi-lingual elderly. *International Journal of Geriatric Psychiatry*, 15(11), 1021–1027.

Chapter 12. A Segue Sideways

1. Yale, R. & Kaplan, D. (2006) Memory loss support groups for residents of assisted living: Enhancing quality of care and quality of life. *Alzheimer's Care Quarterly*, 7(4), 226–242.

Chapter 13. Pilot Project Evaluation

1. Clare, L., Linden, D., Woods, R., Whitaker, R., Evans, S., Parkinson, C., van Paasschen, J., Nelis, S., Hoare, Z., Yuen, K., & Rugg, M. (2010). Goal-oriented cognitive rehabilitation for people with early-stage Alzheimer disease: A single-blind randomized controlled trial of clinical efficacy. *American Journal of Geriatric Psychiatry*, 18(10), 928–939.

2. Law, M., Baptiste, S., Carswell, A., et al. (2005). *Canadian Occupational Performance Measure* (Fourth Edition). Ottawa, ON: CAOT Publications ACE.

3. Georgia Health Policy Center. (2012). *A (Draft) Report of Findings for the Early-Stage Alzheimer's Clinical Counseling Program*. Atlanta, GA: Georgia Division of Aging Services.

4. Personal correspondence (in clinical consultation sessions) with project counselors Suzette Binford, Susan Formby, and Janice Adams.

Chapter 14. Denouement: Fitting It All Together

1. Eliot, T.S. (1942). *Little Gidding/Four Quartets*. London: Faber.

2. Lamott, A.

INDEX